# The Garden of Eden Molecule

# The Garden of
# Eden Molecule

## The Key to Youth,
## Health and Longevity

*Ronald Kotulak*
*Donna Kotulak, Editor*

Writer's Showcase
San Jose  New York  Lincoln  Shanghai

The Garden of Eden Molecule
The Key to Youth, Health and Longevity

Writer's Showcase
an imprint of iUniverse.com, Inc.

For information address:
iUniverse.com, Inc.
5220 S 16th, Ste. 200
Lincoln, NE 68512
www.iuniverse.com

ISBN: 0-595-13848-9

Printed in the United States of America

# Contents

# *Introduction*

People today can look forward to the longest and healthiest life spans the world has ever known. An astonishing 62-percent increase in life expectancy since the turn of the 20th century has given Americans 30 more years in the blink of an eye. And we continue to grow younger; the average life expectancy is 76 years and is climbing at the rate of seven hours a day. This trend contradicts the old notion that we are given a fixed number of years and no more—and indicates that life span is extremely malleable and will continue to be extended indefinitely.

An even more spectacular trend—living to a healthy, productive old age that is capped by a swift death—is making second, third and fourth careers increasingly common. A growing number of people are living 99.9 percent of their lives free of chronic diseases and dying abruptly in old age without suffering the long, lingering illnesses that have plagued previous generations and that were once considered the inevitable burden of old age.

The payoff from a healthy lifestyle is obvious. Dr. James F. Fries of Stanford University has been following graduates of the University of Pennsylvania for more than three decades. In 1980 Fries created a controversy by challenging the assumption that all people will be struck by disease and disability as they grow old. Critics scoffed at his contention that healthy living could prevent the downward spiral. Fries now has the strongest evidence to date showing that healthy habits prevent disabilities.

His Pennsylvania graduates started out even: all were healthy, all came from the same socioeconomic background and all had equivalent educational experiences. But by the time they reached their 70s, they were very different. Those who became obese, ate few fruits or vegetables, smoked 30 or more cigarettes a day or got no regular vigorous exercise were laid low with numerous disabilities, while those who didn't have these risk factors were healthy and vigorous. The men in the high-risk group had a 50 percent higher death rate and a 100 percent greater disability rate than males in the low-risk group.

Seeing more and more people avoid chronic sickness and disability until the last few weeks or months of life is dramatically changing our perception of aging. Instead of dreading growing old, we can look forward to a vigorous new period of life that humans have never experienced before. As the 76 million baby boomers, America's most educated and healthiest generation, move into old age, they will plow aside many of the infirmities that were once considered normal.

Scientists are turning the tables on evolution to make aging as controllable as planning a career. They are figuring out the biology of aging from studying the free radical, the Adam and Eve molecule. Free radicals, which date back to the beginning of time, play two opposing roles, giving life and taking it. Free radicals supply us with the energy we need to live, but they also randomly and gradually destroy the genes and cellular machinery of our bodies to produce wrinkles, cancer, dementia and the many other manifestations of aging. **All chronic diseases, from heart disease to diabetes to Alzheimer's disease, are free radical diseases.**

"We're learning what it takes to live longer," says Dr. Maria Fiatrone, chief of the Exercise Physiology Laboratory at the USDA's Human Research Center for Aging at Tufts University. "If we could put all of it together in one package, we'd all probably live to our maximum life expectancy, around 100 years."

In 1990, Fiatrone exploded the myth that loss of muscle and bone in the frail elderly was irreversible. Using resistance training, Fiatrone was able to build up muscle strength in nursing home patients in their 80s and 90s. Instead of being doomed to spend the rest of their lives in wheelchairs or in bed, they were able to get around on their own again. For Fiatrone's elderly, who were about as sedentary and old as human beings could be, the exercise program produced wondrous results, proving that at any age there's a lot of room for improvement. If a person can increase muscle strength at age 99 by 100 to 200 percent, it means that a lot of what we think of as aging is simply disuse.

Just as Fiatrone is highlighting the effects of strength-building exercise on health and aging, T. Colin Campbell, a Cornell University nutritional biochemist, is underscoring the benefits of a good diet. In a unique study called the China Project, Campbell is showing which foods are the most healthful and which are most harmful. The big difference in the diets in different Chinese provinces is the amount of fat they contain, ranging from 6 percent of total calories to a high of 24 percent. In the U.S., by comparison, fat intake ranges from a low of 25 percent of calories to more than 50 percent.

Cancer is a local disease in China, compared with the U.S., where it is more a national disease. Cancer rates in China vary by several hundred percent between provinces, whereas U.S. rates among the states vary by no more than 20 to 30 percent. "The big story coming out of the China study is that as soon as we start putting animal foods in our diet in place of plant foods, we get into trouble. Period. It's that simple," Campbell insists.

But the biology of this phenomenon is extraordinarily complex. Basically, what's present in plant foods tends to protect people against degenerative diseases, while what's present in animal foods tends to worsen these conditions. "There are areas in China where cancer and heart disease are virtually unknown," Campbell says. "That tells us that, in theory, if we just knew what in the world these plant foods are doing, people in the U.S. could get close to zero in some of these degenerative diseases, at least up to the age of 75 or 80."

Campbell's mystery is now being solved by scientists who are discovering what it is in food that serves as an antidote to aging—the antioxidant, which plays a vital role in keeping damage from free radicals under control. The antioxidant is the Garden of Eden molecule. It is safe to say that the increasing consumption of antioxidants over the past four decades is a major factor in the continuing extension of life span, the decline in free radical diseases and plummeting disability rates. One out of two Americans now takes antioxidant supplements. And we are finding a gold mine of antioxidants all around us in the fruits and vegetables we eat.

*The Garden of Eden Molecule* explains how people who have adopted healthy lifestyles—eating plenty of fruits and vegetables, exercising regularly and shunning high-fat foods and cigarettes, for example—are maintaining a positive balance between antioxidants and free radicals. They are the people who are most likely to use education to their advantage, compressing illness, if they do get sick, into the shortest possible time before death. The brain is our most important anti-aging organ—the more you know, the wiser your lifestyle choices. And the more education you have, the longer you can expect to live in a state of good health. A study of nearly 140,000 Americans, whose average age is 73, shows that those with more than 12 years of education have a much longer life and a better quality of life up until the very end than people who have eight years or fewer of education. Simply put, education beyond high school adds a decade or more of youth and health to your life.

**At no time in history have scientists been so close to understanding aging. Far from being an unfathomable mystery, aging is turning out to be something simple and basic—the result of the interplay between free radicals, with their life-giving and life-taking properties, and antioxidants, which determine which of these properties, the giving or the taking, prevails at any given time.**

Until recently, there were nine distinct theories of aging. One by one, they have become explainable as the consequence of free radical damage, making the free radical theory the grand unified theory of aging. Scientific evidence continues to confirm it.

*The Garden of Eden Molecule* has a clear message—the more we know about how and why we age, the more we can control our fate. We have far more to say about how long we live than do our genes. Each day, the choices we make, the things we do and the foods we eat enable us to adjust the ratio of antioxidants to free radicals, tipping the balance heavily in our favor.

# 1

# The Free Radical:
# The Adam and Eve Molecule

"My father died of a heart attack at 64. Why did he have coronary artery disease? He had a lousy lifestyle. He smoked a lot. When you smoke you put in carbon monoxide, which increases your body's free radical generation. He also ate a very high-fat diet. So he was putting in huge amounts of free radicals and mutating himself. To me, that is as straightforward and logical as it could possibly be."

Looking back on his father's untimely death through the cell-piercing eyes of a molecular biologist, Douglas Wallace can see now that his father burned his biological candle at both ends. His explanation of the new knowledge about the molecular science of aging was bittersweet: "I wish my dad had known about free radicals."

Wallace, of Emory University, belongs to a new breed of scientists. Armed with a dazzling array of discoveries, these researchers believe they are at last on the threshold of learning nature's deepest secrets—why there is life, why we age and why we get sick. They are piecing together the story of how a spark of nature's fire billions of years ago has become the free radical of today, the giver and sustainer of life. Without free radicals, life as we know it could not exist.

But we pay a price for their precious gift of life: free radicals are the reason we age and get sick. They give us wrinkled skin, hardened arteries, clouded eyes, dulled brains, cancerous cells and, over time, charred residue in every organ, bone and joint.

Virtually unknown until relatively recently, free radicals—also referred to by such unglamorous names as unpaired electrons and reactive oxygen species—form the basis of a profound, new understanding of disease. With this knowledge, researchers are already devising ways to prevent and cure cancer, heart disease and Alzheimer's disease. And they boldly proclaim that they can make people live longer and healthier.

Similar scientific leaps have been made in the past to improve the human condition. The discovery in 1742 that eating limes could prevent scurvy forged the concept that critical nutrients, such as vitamin C, are essential for warding off certain diseases. Pasteur's monumental finding in the 1850s that germs cause infection led to improved hygiene, sterilization, sanitation, immunization and antibiotics. More recently, scientists in the 1970s showed that mutated genes increase susceptibility to cancer and other diseases.

But these accomplishments pale in comparison with the revolution in biology now taking place. Driven by the powerful tools of molecular biology and genetic engineering, the revolution promises to dramatically change the way we look at life itself. The study of free radicals goes to the heart of the disease process, exposing its basic mechanism to explain how genes get mutated and acquire their ominous, illness-inducing characteristics.

"Many, many diseases have a component of free radical damage," explains Balz Frei, an Oregon State University biochemist who is tracking the link between free radicals and coronary artery disease. "It may not always be the most important thing, but somewhere along the line, free radical damage always seems to play a role, either a causative role or an exacerbating role."

Free radicals occupy a very special place in the scheme of things—they are the force that brings atoms and molecules together. If there's anything nature abhors more than a vacuum, it's a lonely electron. If electrons were happy being by themselves, the universe would be a cold, dark, still place. Just as most people who get divorced yearn to be married again, electrons have a desperate need to couple and when they do, they provide the fire-works that breathe life into inanimate objects.

The free radical is the Adam and Eve molecule in the sense that it gives life but also takes it away, like Adam and Eve, who had it all but lost it. In the Bible story, God created Adam out of dust by blowing the breath of life into him. Modern science now understands that breath to be the free radical. Free radicals are also the very essence of aging. For all living organisms, free radicals are tantamount to time itself, our biological clocks; they are the molecular seconds that inexorably tick away, defining our beginning and end. After we die, the free radicals in us move on to perform their chemical magic elsewhere.

When free radicals are good, they are very, very good. With their energy-inducing power, free radicals enable the molecules that make up chemicals, which by themselves can do nothing, to build the genes that all living things depend on and the chemistry that makes the genes work. In existence since the beginning of time, perhaps 15 billion years, free radicals are in our eyes, ears and brains, enabling us to see, hear and think. Free radicals are one of the body's chief weapons for destroying germs. Their ability to deliver quick hits and then vanish enables cells to use them to deliver rapid messages, telling blood vessels to relax, for example, and enhancing communication between brain cells.

But when free radicals are bad, they're awfully bad. They are all around us—causing metals to rust, sliced apples to turn brown, meat to spoil, bread to toast, skin to sunburn and curtains to fade in sunlight. Cigarette smoke teems with free radicals, accounting for one of three cancer cases and one of four cases of heart disease in the U.S. But by far the majority of the free radicals that batter us are made in our own cells. We don't rust like metal, but our flesh undergoes the same kind of radical terrorism that iron does when exposed to the elements. Premature babies are the first to be scorched by free radicals; they are born before their antioxidant shield is developed enough to protect them from the onslaught of free radicals that prematurity induces. The resulting damage can produce epilepsy and other neurological and physical abnormalities.

In its drive to pair up with another electron, a free radical has the nasty habit of stealing an electron from a complacent molecule. Such thievery damages the molecule and turns it into a ferocious free radical that goes on the prowl to steal an electron from another molecule. This chain reaction of free radical production harms flesh and bone. Free radicals tear at genes to cause mutations and cancer, they riddle cells in the lining of arteries to induce heart disease and they set land mines that shatter brain cells, producing the memory loss characteristic of Alzheimer's disease and other neurodegenerative disorders. In short, free radicals can cause so many things to go wrong with us that they are largely responsible for our modern epidemic of lifestyle killers.

By studying how these red-hot rivets destroy the magnificent structures they have helped build, researchers are uncovering answers to some of the great mysteries of biology. Dr. Denham Harman of the University of Nebraska College of Medicine uncovered the first clue to exactly when the free radical clock started to tick. As a physician and biochemist, Harman was intrigued by the possibility that there might be something so essential that it could give life and take it away. In 1954, he came up with the free radical theory of aging. "It is remarkable that life, with its beautiful order, may owe its origin to and be sustained by a class of chemical reactions whose outstanding characteristic is their unruly nature," Harman says.

**In essence, the free radical theory states that aging is the haphazard accumulation of harmful changes in the body produced by free radicals. The more free radicals a person makes, the faster his or her flesh, brain and bones deteriorate and the faster he or she will age. The most significant contribution of the theory is the discovery that aging can be modified—dramatically slowed down or speeded up.**

Harman's new understanding of aging was considered outlandish at first and was dismissed by his scientific peers. Anyone who embraced it was laughed at. Daniel L. Gilbert and Rebeca Gerschman ran into opposition in the mid 1950s when they proposed that oxygen was a poison that damaged cells by producing free radicals. It was, they said, the same kind of damage caused by X-rays and other forms of radiation. They called oxygen a very unusual poison, different from any other because it's also the energy of life. "People didn't want to hear that. They were ridiculing the idea," recalls Gilbert.

The atmosphere we breathe is 20 percent oxygen. If it were 100 percent oxygen, free radicals would chew up our lungs and other organs and we wouldn't survive more than two days. Gilbert's pioneering work on free radicals has now become mainstream science. He heads the Unit on Reactive Oxygen Species established a few years ago by the National Institute on Neurological Disorders and Stroke in acknowledgement of the role that free radicals play in disease. Scientific recognition has also come to Harman, who has been nominated for a Nobel Prize.

It is generally believed that life began spontaneously about three-and-a-half billion years ago by free radicals that randomly kick-boxed chemicals around until a self-replicating molecule—the first gene—took shape. Many copies of that gene could be made and, by breaking the genes apart and rebuilding and rearranging them, free radicals produced genetic mutations that allowed evolution to progress. All life forms today—from bacteria to humans—share genes that originated in that first breath of life.

Having created life, free radicals were then called upon to sustain it. Life remained pretty simple and sluggish until one primitive form of bacteria figured out how to make lots of energy by burning hydrogen from food and oxygen from the atmosphere. Before then, the earliest organisms made free radicals for energy consumption the hard way: without oxygen in the early atmosphere, they had to break down water to make hydrogen, a weak energy source. In this energy-producing process, these primordial organisms expelled oxygen, which gradually built up in the atmosphere and, over time, spelled their doom. Many of the earliest living things were defenseless against the damage from the oxygen-produced free radicals and died off.

But oxygen is also a high-octane fuel and some of the organisms present about three billion years ago evolved the capacity to benefit from its growing supply. They mated oxygen with hydrogen to make water, liberating six times more energy than any other organism was capable of doing. With this newfound energy, organisms that had barely gotten by with one cell or just a few cells could grow enormously bigger and fantastically diverse. They could even develop brains. It took time to get the genetic blueprints just right, but that's exactly what happened in the Cambrian explosion some 650 million years ago, when a vast multitude of life forms sprang into existence.

The bacteria that started the energy splurge had found a way to package the energy inherent in free radicals into a safe molecule called adenosine triphosphate (ATP). It was a hand grenade of energy that could be used anywhere in the bacterial cell to run enzyme reactions, repair DNA, provide locomotion and drive other vital activities. This energy system was so good that all the other bacteria wanted it. So they did what bacteria did then and still do—they swallowed the energy-producing bacteria, advancing evolution by whole cells rather than by single-gene mutations.

It was a good deal for all. The swallowing bacteria were infused with invigorating new energy to play the survival-of-the-fittest game. The swallowed bacteria found safe homes where they didn't have to worry about finding food or fighting off predators. The ATP packets of energy-producing genes maintained their independence, remaining, for the most part, outside their host's genes. The symbiotic relationship between the host genes and the captured genes created a living energy machine that made possible the variety and complexity of life we have today.

These energy-producing bacterial genes, called mitochondria, are still around; in fact, they exist by the hundreds in all of our cells. And they still act like bacteria, dividing on their own. Mitochondria's ageless genetic material, or DNA, is separate from the DNA in the cell's nucleus. Mitochondria are passed on to children only from their mothers because mitochondria ride along with an egg when it is fertilized. Sperm, even though they use the energy produced by mitochondria in their frantic, squiggly journey to reach an egg, leave their own mitochondria behind after their DNA has penetrated the egg.

Mitochondria use 85 percent of the oxygen we breathe to make energy. Oxygen molecules burst from our lungs into the bloodstream, which carries them throughout the body. Every day, billions of oxygen molecules are delivered to each of our cells to stoke their mitochondrial free radical furnaces. Some 20 billion free radicals are produced daily in every cell. In one year, the 100 trillion cells in the average human body will have produced five pounds of free radicals—700 million quadrillion of them.

Such enormous numbers are bound to spell trouble. Like sparks flying off a metal grinder, some free radicals get away, leaping out of the frenzied mitochondria, hellish riders on the backs of oxygen molecules. On the loose, free radicals can damage genes and the proteins and fats that make up a cell's structure. By meticulously measuring genetic damage, Bruce Ames of the University of California, Berkeley, has been able to calculate that, on average, the DNA in each cell sustains 10,000 free radical hits per day.

Nature, being well aware of this danger, built in copious repair systems to cut out DNA that is damaged by free radicals and replace it with healthy DNA. But the repair system has an Achilles heel. About one percent of damaged DNA escapes repair and becomes incorporated into a person's genetic code as mutations. Although these mutations can increase a person's risk of cancer and other diseases, they foretell a more sinister fate: as they accumulate, they impair the cells' ability to function, slowly stealing away the time that a person has to live.

Proteins and fats—which form enzymes, cell membranes and other critical structures—are in this mortal struggle between free radical damage and the body's efforts to repair it. Normally, injured proteins are dissolved and new ones built to replace them, a repair process that is especially vital for brain and muscle cells. But under constant harassment by free radicals, the system is gradually disabled. Broken and fractured proteins go unrepaired and the cells that house them cannot work anymore.

In the end, the carnage is gruesome. By age 80, we are all carrying around a tremendous burden of splintered and non-working proteins. According to Earl Stadtman, a cell biologist at the National Heart, Lung and Blood Institute, about 40 percent of the proteins that give us form and function are irreversibly damaged by that age. The residue of free radical damage is what we call aging, which we see, for example, in wrinkles, sagging skin, failing eyesight and lack of energy. Organs that produce hormones are one of the biggest victims of free radical damage. As hormones decline, brain cells wither, muscles atrophy and bones disintegrate. Bruce Ames sees a similar desolate picture for genes. In old age, the DNA in each human cell, he estimates, has about two million permanent mutations, making its genetic blueprint increasingly unreadable.

With a mutation rate 10 times higher than that of the main DNA in the nucleus of a cell, mitochondria melt down, accelerating the aging process. As their genetic damage rapidly increases, mitochondria spew out increasing numbers of blistering free radicals. Mitochondria basically destroy themselves; without their ability to produce energy, their human host runs out of steam.

"If you ask old people what their problem is, it's that they don't have any more energy," observes mitochondria expert Doug Wallace. "It's harder to get up. It's harder to walk. It's harder to do everything. They get tired all the time. They've been telling us that for 10,000 years. Why can't we accept that as a real observation?"

Organs are affected by free radical damage at different rates, depending on how much mitochondria energy they use. The brain is often the first organ to start failing because it requires the most energy to function. (Next in line are the heart, muscles, kidneys, hormone system and liver.) Looking for the extent of free radical damage to mitochondria in the aging human brain, neurologist M. Flint Beal of Massachusetts General Hospital and Harvard Medical School found that the damage in the autopsied brains of people older than 70 was 15 times greater than that in the brains of people younger than 50. For Alzheimer's patients, the situation was even worse—three times more free radical damage to their mitochondria than that found in the brains of people the same age who had died of other causes, or 45 times greater than that found in younger people.

In the near future, people may be able to learn how quickly or slowly they are aging, or if they are getting Alzheimer's or some other disease, simply by testing their urine or blood for signs of free radical damage. Such tests can tell us when we need to take measures to limit the danger from excessive oxidation. Free radical damage to fats, which help make up the membranes of cells, can already be measured in urine or blood. In repairing injury to their membranes, cells cut out fats that have been charred by free radicals and replace them with healthy fats. The debris from this repair work, which is washed away in the blood and then in the urine, contains the fingerprints of free radical damage, chemicals called isoprotanes.

Garrett Fitzgerald of the University of Pennsylvania in Philadelphia and his colleagues tested the urine of smokers and found that it contained much higher levels of isoprotanes than the urine of nonsmokers. Cigarette smoke fills the lungs with unleashed free radicals, which course through the blood, damaging cells throughout the body.

Alzheimer's disease is thought to be the result of free radical damage to brain cells, caused primarily by the many forms that inflammation can take in the brain. Checking urine levels of isoprotanes, researchers found that they were higher in people who had been diagnosed with Alzheimer's disease than in healthy older people. The ability to measure brain cell destruction in people with Alzheimer's disease will help physicians to determine which therapies work best to curb the disease.

Our rate of aging may also be determined by a simple test that measures the rate of free radical wear and tear on our genes. Using a chip about the size of a business card, University of Wisconsin scientists can examine 6,000 genes at a time. The chip contains DNA sequences that match the sequences of specific genes in a cell; the genes can then be plucked out of the cell and studied. When these genes are examined, chemical subunit by chemical subunit, the telltale signs of free radical damage stand out clearly.

Studying cells swabbed from the inside of the mouth or from a drop of blood, the chips make it possible to determine whether a person is aging too fast, at just the right rate or, even better, slowly. Such a genetic test will also measure the anti-aging effects of diet, exercise and other strategies. With this new ability to easily monitor the rate at which you are aging, you will be able to manipulate it on a daily basis.

While people generally experience similar symptoms of aging, the damage from free radicals occurs sooner in some and later in others. Individual body parts also age at different rates, depending on the degree of havoc caused by free radicals. "Free radical damage is indiscriminate," says Stadtman. "Free radicals will damage whatever they're close to. The evidence that proteins, fats and DNA are damaged is formidable. There's no question that all of these compounds are harmed under conditions of oxidative stress and even under normal conditions of free radical production. Aging is the result of the loss of the mechanisms that repair that damage."

If loss of repair produces such dire consequences, why does nature allow it to take place? One reason is that repair is as good as it needs to be to ensure that an organism produces offspring, sending genes on their never-ending quest for the future. After the reproductive years, nature doesn't care much what happens to an organism. Another reason is that, while most genetic mutations are bad for an organism because they are the harbingers of disease and aging, some mutations may endow an organism with new skills for survival.

Gene mutations are the architects of evolution, but they are also the demons of aging. The molecular clock that leads to the decline in all of us is not programmed in our genes. It is driven by random free radical hits to our DNA, primarily the critical 16 genes that make up the energy-producing mitochondria in each of our cells. People die of different diseases, but the diseases are all linked to misfiring mitochondria.

Mitochondria are the epicenter of the aging process. We are born with mitochondria that range from very bad to very good. If your mitochondria are bad and they produce a lot of free radicals, you mutate faster and you start getting all of the chronic diseases of aging early in life. An extreme example of the effects of mutated mitochondria are people with a syndrome called myoclonic epilepsy and ragged red fiber disease (MERRF); their mitochondria produce only one-fourth as much energy as normal mitochondria do and they leak excessive amounts of free radicals. As a result, people with the disorder age rapidly, developing heart disease, diabetes and dementia in their 20s and 30s and dying prematurely.

People who are born with very good mitochondria, on the other hand, have a lot of energy, their free radical production is low and they tend to live into their 90s in good health. But even good mitochondria can't protect against the effects of unhealthy habits that promote free radical generation, such as cigarette smoking, excessive alcohol consumption, a high-fat diet and too little exercise.

Another bad habit that can hasten aging is depriving yourself of sleep. As scientists discover the biological reasons for why we need sleep, they are finding that sleep is as essential to good health as exercise and a nutritious diet. Sleep deprivation, in addition to shortchanging brain cells of much-needed energy, sets in motion hormonal imbalances that can physically etch away the brain and its functions, like a free radical acid. Lack of sleep increases levels of the potentially harmful stress hormone cortisol, which can generate free radicals when it gets out of hand. Brain images of people with abnormally high cortisol levels reveal shrinkage in areas of their brains, particularly the hippocampus, a primary organizer of learning and memory.

How quickly a whole population can increase free radical production, age rapidly and die early has been vividly demonstrated in Russia. Between 1984 and 1987, things were going relatively well—life expectancy rose 3.2 years for men (to 64.9 years) and 1.2 years for women (to 74.3 years). But with the chaotic dissolution of the Soviet Union, life became harsh for vast numbers of Russians. To cope, many started drinking heavily and smoking. Their nutrition worsened as they ate more high-fat foods and fewer vegetables and fruits. They were riddling their bodies with free radicals at a frenetic pace. The destruction to their bodies revealed itself between 1987 and 1994 with a sharp decline in life expectancy—by 7.3 years for men and 3.3 years for women.

This lesson was not lost on Doug Wallace, the scientist who saw how free radicals shortened his father's life. If Wallace had known then what he knows now, he would have told his father that he could stop "mutating" himself and live longer. "All you have to do is stop smoking, keep your weight down, exercise regularly and eat a low-fat, high-antioxidant diet. Then you'll eliminate the free radicals that cause mutations." He might also advise his father to take daily antioxidant supplements like the ones he takes himself: vitamins A, C, D and E and the B-complex vitamins, including folate.

# 2

# The Antioxidant:
# The Garden of Eden Molecule

So strong is the desire to stay young that some people have undergone testicle transplants from adolescent monkeys, transfused themselves with new blood and swallowed all kinds of bitter potions. Now, thousands of scientists from university, government and pharmaceutical laboratories are racing to develop what they believe will be the first true elixirs of youth. They are finding that most of the different roads they are taking in search of ways to understand and slow aging lead to the same destination—free radicals and antioxidants, the yin and yang of life.

The antioxidant is the Garden of Eden molecule, the closest thing we have to the Garden's tree of life. Its fruit was to provide Adam and Eve with immortality, had they not been expelled from Paradise for eating the forbidden apple, which they had been told would make them godlike. Thousands of different antioxidants exist in the fruits and vegetables we eat today, providing us, if not with immortality, at least with the opportunity for a longer and healthier life. Antioxidants are on the prowl everywhere in the body, disarming free radicals before they can do harm.

No goal is more important in biology today than learning how antioxidants work, where they come from and how they can be enhanced. Such knowledge could have a greater impact on our lives than any other medical advance, including the development of antibiotics and vaccines. Emboldened by wonderful new discoveries, especially in

17

the last few years, researchers are closing in on the secret of how and why we age. They are also learning what it is about the delicate balance between antioxidants and free radicals that predisposes us to chronic diseases.

Free radicals are like smoke that pollutes the air when coal is burned to generate electricity. As we now require scrubbers on smokestacks to reduce air pollution, nature has devised many types of antioxidants to stop free radicals in their tracks. Without antioxidants, free-radical-driven processes such as cancer could not be kept at bay. Free radicals and antioxidants are constantly at war and, for the most part, they cancel each other out.

Antioxidants are at their best early in life, allowing babies to grow up to be healthy adults. But, like a gambling casino where the odds always favor the house if you play long enough, the balance between antioxidants and free radicals eventually tips in favor of free radicals. Free radicals that are not arrested and disarmed by antioxidants can cause mutations in genes, which can lead to cancer. And they can damage critical enzymes and cell structures to produce heart disease and neurological disorders. At first, the damage caused by free radicals is manageable. Your body's own repair mechanisms clip out mutated genes and replace them with healthy ones. Cell membranes and internal structures that have been burned and charred by free radicals are removed and new replacement parts constructed and fitted into place.

At some point (most people notice it around middle age), the biological clock starts to run faster. Just as desperate gamblers raise their bets in an attempt to recoup their losses, mitochondria, the power plants in cells, work overtime in a struggle to keep energy flowing. As they do, they generate free radicals in unprecedented numbers. The ensuing damage piles up, challenging the body's superb biological machinery. Finally, raging free radicals can destroy the mitochondria themselves, cutting off the body's energy supply. It is this final blow that doctors euphemistically call "death from natural causes."

Despite the increasing evidence that mitochondria injury increases with age, there is growing hope that the future can be changed. "We're finally at the point of being able to identify the key members of the antioxidant defense system," says cell biologist Tory Hagen of the University of California at Berkeley, who has shown that old mitochondria can be rejuvenated. "By enhancing antioxidant activity through dietary means and supplements, we may be able to restore some of the ability of the mitochondria to meet their cellular energy demands. It's beginning to look as though we can affect a lot of these age-related phenomena."

**Of all the theories of aging that have been proposed, only the free radical theory is solid enough to be tested in the laboratory. In its elementary form, the theory says that aging is the result of the haphazard accumulation of free radical damage to genes and cells. Therefore, aging can be retarded by reducing free radical damage—either by increasing antioxidant levels or by reducing the body's production of free radicals. Scientists now have direct evidence that both processes— increasing antioxidants and decreasing free radical production—can indeed slow aging.**

The new discoveries are also making it clear that people can already do a lot for themselves to retard aging. "If people ate healthy diets, didn't smoke and exercised, they would be doing 90 percent of what is possible to do right now to minimize their risk of developing the major diseases that cause most people in our society to die," according to Dr. James Mulshine of the National Cancer Institute's Biomarkers and Prevention Research Branch, which is studying the molecular basis of disease.

The reasoning is compelling. Fruits and vegetables are filled with natural antioxidants, smoking is a major source of free radicals and exercise helps cells defend themselves against the ravages of free radicals. Underscoring the importance of this advice are the results of a nationwide study of the eating habits of more than 42,000 women. Women who eat more fruits and vegetables, which are loaded with antioxidants, reduce their risk of dying of all causes by 30 percent. And it takes only a small increase in the consumption of these foods each week to decrease the risk of dying of cancer, heart attack and stroke.

Almost every part of the body, from the skin to the brain, now appears to be protected by antioxidants. Even our lungs get a second wind from these free-radical fighters. Cornell University scientists, looking at tens of thousands of adults in the U.S. and China, found that people who have the highest levels of antioxidants, such as selenium and vitamins C and E, in their blood have far better lung function than people with the lowest levels. The antioxidant-rich people got their antioxidants from eating plenty of fruits and vegetables and taking vitamin supplements.

High levels of antioxidants may even help prevent asthma, emphysema and chronic bronchitis, as well as protect some smokers from lung damage known as chronic obstructive pulmonary disease. When the Cornell researchers measured lung power, they were stunned to find that, compared with nonsmokers who have high antioxidant levels, the nonsmokers with below-average antioxidant levels have lung function similar to that of a person who has smoked a pack of cigarettes a day for 10 years.

One of the first clues to the importance of antioxidants came from the laboratory of Michael Rose at the University of California, Irvine, in experiments on fruit flies. His idea was to create population pressures that would push hidden longevity genes to the forefront. By allowing only those eggs laid by the oldest fruit flies to hatch generation after generation, he found that these offspring lived longer and longer. Since 1980, when Rose began his experiment, he has bred fruit flies that live twice the normal fruit-fly life span. What is the secret? Robert Tyler, also at Irvine, found that the long-lived fruit flies have a souped-up version of a gene that makes the antioxidant superoxide dismutase (SOD). The evolutionary pressure to which Rose subjected the flies favored the emergence of a powerful antioxidant gene, which protected them from free radical damage.

In 1990, another gene, called Age-1, took center stage. Thomas Johnson of the University of Colorado at Boulder found that a mutation in the Age-1 gene doubled the life span of the tiny, dirt-dwelling worm, C. elegans. Mutations can cause genes to overproduce or underproduce proteins. The worms that were defying aging had mutated Age-1 genes that were overproducing SOD and perhaps another natural antioxidant, catalase, giving them the upper hand in their battle against free radicals.

Scientists at the University of California at San Francisco, headed by Dr. Charles Epstein, genetically engineered mice to have an extra copy of the SOD gene in every cell. With high hopes that the mice would live longer, the scientists eagerly watched and waited as the animals grew older. But instead of breaking longevity records, the transgenic mice were dying off at the same rate as normal mice. The scientists weren't disappointed for long, however, because something mysterious had happened: the genetically altered animals had become supermice—they could deflect stresses that would cause free radical damage in normal mice.

"The extra SOD gene protected these mice from almost any bad thing you could do to them," marvels Epstein. "We gave them strokes, acute trauma and toxic drugs and they were protected."

Still, the scientists were puzzled about why the extra SOD gene didn't help the mice live longer. Were they on the wrong track? The mystery was solved in 1994 in an experiment by molecular biologists Rajindar S. Sohal and William C. Orr of Southern Methodist University. It would be the first proof of the free radical theory of aging—that increasing antioxidants subdues free radicals and slows aging.

The Texas scientists had been putting human antioxidant genes—SOD or catalase—into fruit flies one at a time. At first, they had the same discouraging results as the California researchers. Each time they gave flies an extra antioxidant gene, the flies developed better protection against free radicals but didn't live longer. A breakthrough came, however, when they gave the fruit flies both human antioxidant genes at the same time. Together, the two genes slowed the aging process in the flies and allowed them to live considerably longer—a 34-percent increase in life span. In human terms, this is like enabling each of us to live 100 years or more.

The flies with the two extra antioxidant genes had significantly lower levels of free radical damage than normal flies. The extra supply of antioxidants mopped up the free radicals before they could cause harm. "We have controlled the rate of aging," Sohal beams. "We haven't abolished the aging process; eventually the transgenic flies slow down, just as regular flies do. But their youthful period lasts longer. As the flies with the extra genes grow older, they are much more active than the others and they are much more robust. This is not only an extension of the length of time that they live, but an improvement in the quality of life as well."

Why were the two antioxidant genes, SOD and catalase, together able to extend life while neither one alone could? In essence, a two-step process is required to quench the fierce free radical superoxide. SOD converts superoxide into hydrogen peroxide, which still possesses free radical activity. Catalase neutralizes this free radical activity by converting hydrogen peroxide into water.

Then came the second proof of the free radical theory—that decreasing free radical production slows aging. Genetic engineers at Massachusetts General hospital demonstrated this with the discovery of a gene called daf-2 that, when mutated, enables C. elegans worms to live two to three times longer than the usual 14 days. In its normal form, daf-2 kicks in when no food is available, causing the tiny worms to go into a state of hibernation. In this state, C. elegans live longer, awakening when their favorite food, soil bacteria, is again available. Hibernation is a common strategy used by animals and insects to survive cold weather, droughts or lack of food. In all of these cases, metabolism slows down and reproduction halts, drastically lowering the need for food. At the same time, free radical production is slowed, effectively suspending the aging process.

Daf-2's most important job is to make an organism's metabolism more efficient, which curbs the production of free radicals. When the Massachusetts General scientists caused a slight mutation in the daf-2 gene, it slowed the metabolism of the worms and dramatically lengthened their life span. The mutation bypassed hibernation, enabling the worms to convert more food into fat, which could be stored for future use. In the process, their cells slowed their combustion of food into energy, which protected the cells from free radical damage. Humans have their own version of the daf-2 gene, which regulates insulin, which in turn regulates metabolism and the production of free radicals.

"How fast we age may be intimately connected to how we burn the calories we eat," says Massachusetts General Hospital's Gary Ruvkun, a molecular geneticist. "Such a correlation of metabolism with longevity supports the free radical theory of aging—free radicals are produced as a natural byproduct of normal metabolism and it is those inevitable destructive molecules that lead to aging."

As molecular biology reveals these crucial steps in the aging process, scientists are developing compounds that may be able to slow it. First on the list are antioxidant supplements, some derived from plants and others made synthetically. You may have to consume some antioxidants in amounts not normally obtainable through the diet in order to get their strongest protection. Dr. Simin Nikbin Meydani and her colleagues at the Nutritional Immunology Laboratory at the Jean Mayer USDA Human Nutrition Research Center on Aging at Tufts University discovered that vitamin E can reverse many of the age-related declines in the immune system, but only at a level of 400 international units (IUs) each day, an amount significantly higher than the level of the vitamin found in the typical diet and much higher than the recommended daily allowance (RDA).

Vitamin E has a strong effect on the immune system's T cells, perking them up so that they can fight viral infections and kill small cancers as quickly as they arise. People in the study who had higher levels of vitamin E had lower rates of infection. Meydani believes that the vitamin works by decreasing free radical damage, thereby giving immune cells a chance to recover and repair themselves to fight again.

Megadoses of some vitamins are being studied to see if they can prevent chronic diseases, but so far the results are inconclusive. From the available evidence, it seems probable that moderate doses may have a major impact against these disorders. This is the approach that the Institute of Medicine, which establishes RDAs, is taking. Recognizing the role that antioxidants play in preventing cell damage from free radicals, the institute recently raised the recommended levels of vitamin E for women by 86 percent and for men by 50 percent. Both women and men should be taking 15 milligrams, or 22 IUs, of vitamin E daily. The recommended upper limit for vitamin E is 1,000 milligrams, or 1,500 IUs.

For vitamin C, the institute has raised the allowance for women by 25 percent and for men by 50 percent. Women should consume 75 milligrams of vitamin C each day and men should consume 90 milligrams. Smokers should add another 35 milligrams a day to these levels because of their increased exposure to free radicals from cigarette smoke. Consuming up to 2,000 milligrams of vitamin C per day appears to be safe. The institute has also established a new RDA for selenium, recommending a daily intake of 55 micrograms for both women and men.

Although antioxidant supplements may retard aging and protect against disease, fruits and vegetables are generally the best sources. Over hundreds of millions of years, plants have evolved thousands of antioxidants to protect themselves against the constant free radical damage they incur from exposure to sunlight. This is why green, leafy vegetables, with large surface areas for absorbing sunlight for photosynthesis, are so rich in antioxidants. When you eat blueberries, strawberries and carrots, you are not only getting vitamins C and E and beta carotene, you are also getting hundreds of other antioxidants, most of which have not yet been identified.

Plant antioxidants are generally referred to as phytochemicals, many of which are pigments that give color to vegetables and fruits. Lutein and other members of the carotene family, for instance, give oranges, summer squash, apricots and peaches their yellow or orange color. The richest sources of lutein are spinach, kale and collard greens, which would be yellow or orange if not for the chlorophyll they contain.

Many plant-based antioxidants have been found circulating in the blood and inside cells, where they mop up free radicals. In the test tube, two thirds of a cup of blueberries has been found to deactivate as many free radicals as do 1,773 IUs of vitamin E and 1,270 milligrams of vitamin

C. Perhaps not every fruit or vegetable packs quite as much protective punch as blueberries, but almost all are good at disarming free radicals.

Lycopene is turning out to be one of the most potent free radical squelchers, far more powerful even than vitamin E. Already associated with a lower risk of some deadly cancers—such as prostate and colon cancer—lycopene has also been found to protect against heart disease. A study of nearly 1,400 European men found that those who consumed the most lycopene in their diet had half the rate of heart disease of men who consumed the least amount of the nutrient. Circulating in the blood, lycopene snuffs out free radicals before they can damage cholesterol and start the buildup of fatty deposits that leads to heart disease.

Lycopene is most abundant in tomatoes, although it is also found in pink grapefruit, watermelon and shellfish such as crab and lobster. Vine-ripened tomatoes have more lycopene than yellow ones or those that ripen after they are picked. Processed tomatoes—such as those found in ketchup, tomato paste and tomato juice—are also good sources of lycopene.

Tomatoes have a long history of improving the health of people all over the world. Italians saw their health take a great leap forward some 500 years ago after Columbus brought tomatoes back from the New World, introducing the red fruit into Italian culinary culture. In addition to lycopene, tomatoes provide folate, vitamins C and A and potassium. In Italy, tomatoes are the second most important source of vitamin C, after oranges. In the United States, tomatoes and tomato-based products are second in popularity only to the potato.

Some antioxidants, such as lutein and zeaxanthin, appear to protect specific organs. For example, lutein and zeaxanthin, members of the carotenoid family, defend the eyes against age-related macular degeneration, a disorder that affects about 13 million Americans and is the major cause of blindness after age 65. The condition results from damage to the macula lutea, a pigmented region of the retina at the back of the eye. The macula lutea contains the highest density of photoreceptors and provides the sharpest vision. When these photoreceptors are damaged, central vision is lost.

Light is necessary for us to see, but it also produces free radicals as it strikes the delicate cells of the eyes. Lutein and zeaxanthin make up the pigment in the macula lutea, providing an antioxidant shield against the excessive onslaught of free radicals that enter the eyes like laser-guided bullets. It's as if nature, realizing how essential light is for vision yet how dangerous it can be, made two antioxidants designed specifically to protect the eyes. They are especially good at filtering out blue light, the most damaging part of the spectrum. The retina is like a curtain on the inside of a window that can fade from sunlight. Just as pulling a shade protects the curtain from free radicals, wearing sunglasses and visors reduces free radical damage to the eyes and lowers the risk of macular degeneration. Cigarette smokers are at increased risk of macular degeneration because cigarette smoke is a major generator of free radicals.

Because the eyes are high on the free-radical hit list, they love antioxidants, whether they come from fruits and vegetables, the best sources, or from supplements. People who eat lots of fruits and vegetables—especially green, leafy vegetables such as spinach, kale and parsley, which are rich in lutein and zeaxanthin—can cut their risk of macular degeneration in half. Other antioxidants, such as vitamins A, C and E, are also protective and have been used to slow the progression of this sight-robbing disorder. Not surprisingly, an adequate supply of antioxidants also dramatically lowers the risk of another eye condition, cataracts, a clouding of the lens of the eye that results from free radical damage from exposure to sunlight and cigarette smoke.

Tufts University researchers have developed a system to measure the ability of different foods to protect cells from free radical damage. According to their system, the ten best free-radical-fighter fruits, starting with the most potent, are prunes, raisins, blueberries, blackberries, strawberries, raspberries, plums, oranges, red grapes and cherries. The top ten vegetables are garlic, kale, spinach, brussels sprouts, alfalfa sprouts, broccoli florets, beets, red bell peppers, onions and corn. The Tufts researchers found that consuming high-ranking fruits and vegetables, such as blueberries and spinach, can raise the antioxidant level in a person's blood by 10 to 25 percent. This wall of protection against free radicals helps to slow the aging process throughout the body, including in the brain, preventing loss of long-term memory and learning and protecting blood vessels from free radical damage.

James Joseph, another Tufts University scientist, never cared much for blueberries, but after seeing how they reverse aging in laboratory rats, he now starts each morning by blending a handful of blueberries into a protein drink. He is convinced it will slow the physical decline that can accompany aging. His research indicates that it's never too late to start: even in old age, antioxidants can help slow the effects of aging. Studying antioxidant-rich fruits and vegetables, he and other researchers have found that giving aging animals extracts of blueberries, strawberries and spinach can dramatically improve their memory. What convinced Joseph to start his daily blueberry diet was seeing that the rats that consumed the equivalent of half a cup of berries daily for eight weeks regained motor skills they had lost as a result of normal aging. Their daily intake of blueberries had reversed the aging process, enabling them to achieve a level of motor proficiency similar to that of much younger rats.

While the protective role of natural antioxidants is becoming more evident, few people get the fullest benefit they should from plant antioxidants. The National Institutes of Health recommends that people eat at least five servings of fruits and vegetables daily, a preventive strategy that more than two-thirds of Americans fail to follow. The five-servings-a-day recommendation is not an arbitrary number: it's the number of servings that gives you the biggest gain with the least effort. Eating more than five servings is even better, but five servings is relatively easy for most of us if we make it a goal and it can greatly improve our health. Eating just one serving (half a cup) of a fruit or vegetable each day reduces your risk of stroke by six percent; eating two servings reduces the risk by 12 percent and each additional serving reduces the risk another six percent; five servings reduce it by 30 percent. Eating more than five servings continues to increase the antioxidant protection against stroke, but not as rapidly as do the first five.

The importance of even a single antioxidant in maintaining life was revealed in 1985 when medical scientists diagnosed the first case of vitamin E deficiency. People with this disorder have a mutation in a gene that is supposed to make a protein that normally extracts vitamin E from food and delivers it into the bloodstream. Without vitamin E to snuff out free radicals, these people quickly develop neurological problems, including slurred speech and loss of muscle control. They are often confined to wheelchairs in their 20s and die in their 30s. "In the last five years we have been giving these people enormous doses of vitamin E," says Dr. Afif Hentati of Northwestern University Medical School. "They're not cured, but they don't get worse."

If the lack of key antioxidants such as vitamin E allows free radicals to swiftly eat away a person's body, then superantioxidants should have the opposite effect, providing the body a coat of armor against free radicals. Robert A. Floyd of the Oklahoma Medical Research Foundation and John Carney of the University of Kentucky showed that an antioxidant called PBN could reverse the effects of aging in gerbils. Older gerbils tend to have twice as much oxidized protein in their brains as younger animals and their ability to learn is only half as good. Floyd and Carney found that repair enzymes, which are designed to remove and replace damaged proteins, also become victims of free radical damage, causing their levels to decline in aging animals.

After giving older gerbils regular injections of PBN over a number of months, the scientists watched as the rate of free radical damage in their brains plummeted and the level of repair enzymes climbed. PBN is believed to specifically protect mitochondria from free radical harm. In a short period of time, the learning and memory capacities of the older animals shot up to the level of the younger ones and stayed there for as long as they were getting PBN.

"It was a surprise to the scientific community and many people refused to believe it at first," says Carney. "It showed that the brain cells were not dead—they just weren't working very well. It means that we can recover some functional status in a system that is greatly impaired but not gone."

Carney's experiment marked the first time that a physiological function—the return of youthful brain function and the restoration of short-term memory—was clearly linked to reducing free radical damage in brain cells. This provided the evidence that it is possible to overcome memory loss with age.

Going a step further, neuroscientist Gary Arendash of the University of South Florida demonstrated that an antioxidant cocktail—PBN and vitamins C and E—when started in late midlife can keep animals in good mental shape as they age. Arendash gave the cocktail treatment to rats that were at an age equivalent to 55 to 60 human years. The treated animals retained their ability to remember and learn while the control animals slipped into mental decline. The mental capacity of the treated rats remained sharp even as they reached an age equivalent to 100 human years. Their control counterparts had died much earlier. When autopsies were performed, the brains of the antioxidant-treated animals were found to have far less free radical damage than those of the controls.

"Our study is encouraging from the standpoint that, if you give antioxidants such as PBN consistently from late middle age on, it could have some real beneficial effects," says Arendash.

While antioxidants such as PBN can reduce free radical injury to mitochondria, Berkeley's Hagen is testing a compound that revives mitochondria that have become listless and inefficient. "This could be a very powerful combination," he says. "Antioxidants could stop the source of free radicals, and other compounds could rejuvenate mitochondria that have already suffered free radical damage." The compound he is testing is called L-acetyl carnitine, or L-car for short. It is a more powerful version of L-carnitine, a natural chemical in our diets found primarily in red meat and dairy products. L-carnitine is used by cells to ferry fats into mitochondria to allow the hydrogen in the fats to be burned with oxygen to produce energy. Some scientists believe that L-car may act as a superantioxidant. However it works, it somehow shakes mitochondria out of their midlife crisis and gets them back to work.

What happens when L-car is given to old animals? It's everyone's dream, according to Hagen. "The old animals that generally just sit there, have no energy, and don't even clean themselves are substantially improved. They have a lot more energy. They're hungrier. They're bouncing around. They're acting very young."

# 3

# *Rejuvenation by Cell Suicide*

If you could collect all the cells in your body that die and are replaced in one year, you'd have a pile that equals another you in terms of volume and weight. That the body has such a fabulous self-renewal system has taken scientists by surprise.

Although they long have known that some cells, such as those in the brains of Alzheimer's patients, die, they viewed such cell death as an enemy of the body. Scientists have also known that some tissues such as skin continuously make new cells and slough off old ones. But they had no notion of the full magnitude of the cell-death-and-rejuvenation process that is now being revealed as an important key to slowing aging and preventing cancer and other diseases.

"Most people tended to think of cell death as some kind of default. Any cell that's unhappy can die—big deal," says geneticist Robert Horvitz of the Massachusetts Institute of Technology and the Howard Hughes Medical Institute, who discovered the first gene that causes cells to die in a purposeful way. "What we found instead was that programmed cell death is a biological process that is every bit as important as cell division and cell differentiation. This has opened people's eyes to a whole new biology."

Poking through the ruins of that enormous pile of cells that we all lose each year, scientists are finding trillions of mistakes—grievous errors that occur in cells and must be eliminated if our bodies are to stay healthy. Most of the mistakes are caused by free radicals. Prior to dying, many of the cells were on their way to becoming cancers and were ordered to kill themselves before they could establish a malignant foothold in the body.

Some had suffered DNA damage from the constant assault of free radicals and were given death sentences when they became dysfunctional or senile.

Other cells—such as white blood cells, which are produced in massive numbers by the immune system to fight infections—die off after they complete their mission. This is what is happening as your swollen lymph glands shrink back to normal when you recover from a respiratory infection; the infection-fighting cells, no longer needed, heed the call to destroy themselves. If they didn't, your body would grow to outlandish proportions with each cold. Other cells die unselfishly after being infected by bacteria or viruses; in dying, the cells deprive the germs of a place to multiply and spread.

**The human body, scientists are finding, comes equipped with an eternal youth program. In theory, if the program worked perfectly, we would not grow older—aging cells would constantly die and be replaced by young, healthy ones. Cell suicide, or programmed cell death, is a biological broom that sweeps our bodies clean of cells that are turning cancerous, aging prematurely, are too severely damaged to function well, or are no longer needed. Scientifically named apoptosis (Greek for falling leaves), the process activates "death" genes, major components of the body's magnificent rejuvenation powers.**

Humans generally find suicide morally repugnant, but our cells have no such qualms. In fact, every one of the 100 trillion cells that give form and function to our bodies contains suicide genes. And most cells—except for those in the brain and heart, where suicide is a no-no—kill themselves when they are damaged or injured to allow the body to replace them with healthy new cells. They either make the decision on their own to commit suicide, or they are given suicide instructions from neighboring cells that sense something is wrong. It's an altruistic response—cells sacrifice themselves for the sake of the whole organism. The goal of apoptosis is to hang on to youth as long as possible, to create a level playing field between old and new, by making sure that old cells die and get out of the way for their youthful replacements.

"Programmed cell death has become the hottest topic in biology because it describes a balance sheet—how to keep the total cell population of the body in check—that we in the scientific community have never dealt with before," says molecular biologist Eugenia Wang of Montreal's McGill University. Wang, who has linked aging to the failure of cells to die when they should, is also director of the Bloomfield Center for Research in Aging at Jewish General Hospital's Lady Davis Institute. "I have not seen a field develop so fast."

Although knowledge about apoptosis is just being uncovered, it is already providing a key to understanding some of life's most fundamental processes. Because nature does not make anything perfect, the machinery that carries out programmed cell death can suffer mortal damage from free radicals over time. The damage can either prevent cells from killing themselves when they should or cause cells to kill themselves when they shouldn't. When injured cells don't commit suicide to make room for the birth of new cells, they grow old and feeble and get put on life support—like Tithonus in Greek mythology, who was granted eternal life but not eternal youth. These dysfunctional cells become the primary sources of aging and cancer.

The opposite is true as well: when free radicals damage genes that regulate cell suicide, they can accelerate cell death. When cells die too fast—that is, when healthy cells commit suicide when they shouldn't—the result can be such devastating degenerative brain disorders as Alzheimer's disease, Parkinson's disease and Huntington's disease.

"I'm optimistic that many of the diseases of old age, and the impact of these diseases, will become less as we understand more about apoptosis," says molecular biologist Judith Campisi of the Berkeley National Laboratory in Berkeley, California. "Maybe we'll still die for the next several generations at 120, or whatever our maximum life span is, but I don't believe we'll spend the last 40 of those years miserable because our bodies are no longer working."

Genes that cause cells to die or that keep them alive are constantly testing each other. They maintain an equilibrium that enables cells to walk a tightrope between continued existence and a quick death. Cell machinery is so complex and so many things can go wrong that our genetic blueprints evolved instructions for cells to destroy themselves whenever they threaten to get out of control. But this tight control over what otherwise would be an unruly mob of cells has a downside: genes that are good for us early in life may be bad for us later on. Genes that protect us from cancer while we're young—such as those that govern DNA repair and programmed cell death—may ultimately cause us to age and develop cancer as we grow older.

Early in life, the body repairs free radical damage to genes swiftly and efficiently. But the repair system itself eventually becomes a victim of free radical damage and loses its power to correct mistakes. At the same time, suicide genes are being hit and crippled by free radicals, impairing the ability of injured cells to die. Damage gradually builds up and the body becomes increasingly populated with undead cells and slips into an aging free-fall that produces wrinkling skin, failing organs and a sputtering immune system. Faced with a steady bombardment of free radicals, some cells may develop a second, deadlier problem—cancer.

Apoptosis is the body's last line of defense against genetic damage and the deterioration that can follow. The body's defenses include antioxidants that extinguish free radicals, mechanisms to repair genetic damage from free radicals, proteins that hold troubled cells together, other proteins that block the replication of mutated genes and programmed cell death when everything else fails. These defenses need to be formidable because free radicals are relentless. And the better these defenses are, the more likely they are to help a person live longer in good health. People who live 100 years or more seem to have better gene-repair systems and superefficient cell-death genes that rid their bodies of enfeebled cells. By destroying damaged, old cells, apoptosis keeps their bodies youthful.

Aging is an integral part of the human experience. But this was not always so. When life began in the form of single cells some four billion years ago, it was immortal. Bacteria, along with humans, are descendents of the first single-cell life forms. Bacteria retain this immortality today: they never die—they just keep dividing. The only things that kill bacteria are starvation or severe injury. When individual cells got together about two billion years ago to form multicell creatures, they traded simplicity and immortality for complexity and the chance to evolve consciousness— the ability of matter to recognize itself. In the process of becoming complex, organisms became mortal. Aging is the price we pay for having brains, hearts and muscles.

Apoptosis is the architect of complexity. During fetal development, programmed cell death eliminates billions of unneeded cells to create a brain and the rest of the human form. Apoptosis lessens the sting of becoming mortal by keeping us in perfect shape for as long as possible, usually until after our reproductive years. But complexity and order have an archenemy—cancer, the constant urge of cells to multiply unchecked, a primordial yearning to reclaim immortality. If not for apoptosis, cancer would have prevented the evolution of higher forms of life.

"Evolution put apoptosis in place to keep us relatively cancer-free until after we have our babies. After about age 50, cancer rates start going up enormously," says Campisi.

Apoptosis at work is not a pretty sight—cells digest themselves. It happens so fast that scientists discovered it only recently. In less than an hour, the suicide program sets in motion processes inside a cell that shrivel its outer membrane, destroy its DNA and set up recycling signs that direct white blood cells to gobble up the debris without leaving a trace. Ironically, cells tagged for death turn to their worst enemy—the free radical—to kill themselves. Dying cells generate copious amounts of free radicals that destroy critical cell structures and hasten the suicide process.

Apoptosis is also a stealthy process, another reason it went unrecognized for so long. When a cell is dying from injury or infection, it sets off an alarm to alert the immune system, provoking inflammation, fever and other noticeable responses. Unlike the immune response, apoptosis silently and imperceptibly disposes of a cell. The process is quick and painless: every six weeks your skin replaces itself, every five days your stomach makes a new lining and every two months your liver replaces all of its cells.

For cells that do not divide very much—such as those in the brain, heart and muscles—we have a different renewal mechanism, which operates under the strict control of survival genes. When the proteins that make up the various parts of brain cells are damaged, they are removed and replaced like old sinks or windows in a house that is constantly under renovation. Within a year, a brain cell can be completely rebuilt from top to bottom, retaining its original appearance and function. Most important, a renovated brain cell keeps what it has learned, just as a house with all new appliances still functions as the same cozy home where you know where everything is. In essence, your body is constantly being remade by apoptosis and renovation. Every year, 98 percent of the atoms that make up your bones, skin, brain, lungs and every other part of your body are removed and replaced with new ones.

Scientists hope that as they learn more about apoptosis, they will be able to solve many other biological riddles. They already have some promising leads:

* Cancer cells appear to spread to other parts of the body and become resistant to chemotherapy and radiation because of a failure of the programmed-cell-death mechanism.

* Aspirin may reduce the risk of colon cancer by triggering the death of precancerous cells.

* The AIDS virus seems able to kill healthy cells of the immune system by sending out chemical messengers that trick white blood cells into committing suicide.

* Viral infections may become persistent because some viruses carry genes that block apoptosis, giving the germs long-term leases in cells where they can grow and multiply.

\*      Secondary damage to cells after a stroke or heart attack results when healthy cells get erroneous signals to kill themselves.

"Apoptosis probably contributes to much more human illness than people have appreciated," according to Dr. Craig Thompson of the University of Chicago. Thompson discovered a gene called bcl-x, which seems to explain how some cells, such as those in the brain, resist cell death, while cells elsewhere in the body welcome it. The bcl-x gene comes in two sizes. The longer version is active in brain cells and protects them from apoptosis. The shorter one is active in cells in which turnover is necessary. "There's going to be a whole new set of medications that will spring up around controlling and regulating cell death," Thompson predicts.

The concept of apoptosis exploded into the scientific community in 1991, when geneticist Horvitz reported the discovery of the first death gene—called ced-3. A year later he found the first anti-death gene—ced-9. Horvitz was intrigued by the microscopic, dirt-loving worm, C. elegans, whose every cell and gene are known, making it a valuable specimen in which to explore the genetic mechanism of apoptosis. After birth, C. elegans grows into an organism of exactly 1,090 cells and then precisely 131 cells die off to form its final shape. (A similar process occurs in humans, for example, during fetal development when the cells that form the webbing between fingers and toes die off to liberate individual digits.) This tightly controlled process occurs in all C. elegans worms. Horvitz found that the cells die when ced-3 increases the production of a chemical messenger of death. The surviving cells contain a larger amount of a life-sustaining chemical produced by ced-9.

The discovery of ced-9 turned out to be a breakthrough as other scientists quickly found a human counterpart to the gene, called bcl-2. Horvitz then showed that the worm ced-9 gene and the human bcl-2 gene were interchangeable. When he knocked out the ced-9 gene in worms, their cells died. When he inserted the human bcl-2 gene into the worms, their cells went on living. The reverse also was found to be true. Ced-9 genes from the worm, placed in human cells grown in test tubes, enabled the human cells to flourish, even after their own bcl-2 genes had been eliminated. Humans and worms diverged hundreds of millions of years ago, yet the genes that control the life and death of their cells remain virtually identical. In fact, the genes have not changed since even before worms and humans went their different ways, attesting to the genes' importance in maintaining the form and function of many-cell creatures.

Is aging inevitable? As new evidence arises to suggest that a reinvigorated cell suicide system can restore some degree of youthfulness, the question becomes pertinent. A new drug, doxazosin, significantly increases apoptosis in older men with enlarged prostates, causing their prostates to shrink to a size similar to that of much younger men and restoring an ease of urinary flow they had lost years earlier. Enlarged prostate, a common ailment of older men, is a typical example of how apoptosis failure can lead to a troublesome pile-up of aged and useless cells.

Berkeley National Laboratory's Campisi found that aged cells accumulate in the basement layer of skin in older people. Careful study of these senescent cells reveals that they become unfriendly. Some of their genes have been damaged by free radicals, causing them to produce dangerous enzymes that degrade collagen and other structural components that give skin its elasticity and suppleness. The evidence suggests that the production of enzymes by damaged cells at least partially explains the form and structure of old skin.

Dr. John Mountz, an immunologist at the University of Alabama at Birmingham, believes that even though immortality is an impossible dream, aging can at least be slowed down. Employing the tools of genetic engineering to give mice an extra copy of a gene that triggers cell death, he has been able to keep the immune systems of old animals acting young. The gene makes a protein, called Fas, that sits on the surface of white blood cells. When white blood cells get too old, or when they have to be pruned back after fighting an infection, messengers alight on the Fas receptors to induce apoptosis.

Over time, however, the Fas receptors become degraded from free radical damage, like deformed locks that no longer permit keys to enter. As a result, white blood cells can no longer receive the messenger of death and they slowly grow older, their power to fight infection declining. Worse, they become confused and quarrelsome. Many scientists now believe that these old white blood cells attack joint tissue to cause rheumatoid arthritis and may cause other autoimmune diseases as well. But the cells in Mountz's mice that were given a double dose of Fas receptors were still able to heed the suicide message and die when they got old and damaged. New white blood cells were born to replace them.

"They look younger," Mountz boasts about his treated mice. "Their coats are nicer looking—they don't have that ratty appearance that old mice get. They don't seem as fat. They have fewer tumors and they live longer. This is a clear demonstration that aging does not have to occur, at least for some parts of the body. There's a lot of vitality that can be maintained just by restoring the normal removal of cells that are nonfunctional."

Centenarians, people who have escaped major aged-related diseases, have superactive immune systems that appear to be renewed much more efficiently than those of people who don't age as well. Perhaps enhancing the cell-death mechanism in people whose own system is inefficient may some day be the standard treatment for rejuvenating us as we age.

*4*

# *Preventing Cancer*

Not long after Joe turned 65, his doctor told him to get his affairs in order; his advanced prostate cancer had failed to respond to any of the traditional treatments. But Joe was reluctant to give up. "I had heard that a low-fat diet might help my kind of cancer," Joe says. "I asked my doctor about it and he threw up his hands and said, 'Go ahead and give it a try. I can't do anything more for you.'"

Joe stuck religiously to vegetables, fruits and grains, eliminating almost all fat from his diet. On a subsequent checkup, his doctor was dumbfounded: Joe's formerly aggressive cancer was in remission. Determined to understand this remarkable turn of events, Joe's physician, Dr. William Fair, chief of urology at the Memorial Sloan-Kettering Cancer Center in New York, began a scientific investigation that ended in his discovery of an important link between fat consumption and the prostate gland: fat generates excessive free radicals by over-heating metabolic processes and the cells that form the prostate are particularly vulnerable to free radical damage.

Joe's case taught scientists an important lesson: reducing free radical stress gives endangered cells an opportunity to rebound. By removing fat from his diet, which had fueled the free radical fireworks inside his body, Joe was giving his prostate a chance to rest and repair itself. And it did. Instead of giving up in defeat, Joe is on the road to recovery.

Although Joe didn't realize it, his low-fat diet tapped into a mother lode of discoveries that are profoundly changing the face of cancer. The revolution in understanding cancer promises to lead to dramatic improvements in ways to prevent and treat this dreaded disease. For many scientists, the new discoveries come as quite a shock. They are finding that much of what they thought they knew about cancer is wrong. Even more disturbing is the fact that cancer cures have not substantially improved in the past five decades. For cancer patients, the discoveries promise new ways to subdue their disease, giving them a second chance. For people who don't have cancer, the findings offer ways to avoid it. The new knowledge will open the door to innovative treatments ranging from such low-tech approaches as a fat-restricted diet to such high-tech solutions as gene therapy.

Until now, cancer treatments have been based on the misconception that uncontrolled cell division is the primary cause of cancer. Previously seen as cancer's Achilles heel, rapid cell proliferation was the main target of treatments, a dogma that has led straight to a dead end. Drugs are used to poison rapidly dividing cells and radiation therapy is given to burn them. The theory behind chemotherapy is that fast-growing cancer cells take up more of the poison than normal cells and die of overdose. Radiation is supposed to be more lethal to the genes of dividing cells than to those of normal cells. Surgery is performed to cut out cancer, but often leaves malignant cells behind.

Dubbed the "poison, burn and slash" approach, these therapies have major drawbacks—they frequently don't work and they produce debilitating side effects because they also destroy healthy cells. Poisoning and burning are effective for some types of cancer but are usually not successful against the tumors that end up killing people, such as cancers of the lung, colon and ovary.

Scientists now believe they know why these often-fatal cancers are resistant to chemotherapy and radiation: they have shut off the body's internal suicide genes, its last defense against cancer. As odd as it seems, damaged genes can build an impenetrable armor against commonly used anticancer therapies. The same kind of genetic damage that deregulates growth-control genes to cause cells to proliferate also can damage the genes that command unhealthy cells to commit suicide. They don't die, no matter how hard they're hit by chemotherapy or radiation. If a genetic mutation blocks apoptosis, compromised cells become undead, like vampires, and their unnatural, immortal state makes them prone to becoming cancerous.

The knowledge that cancer cells have disobeyed their normal genetic instructions to commit suicide is so new that it is just now beginning to trickle into medical schools. It is ushering in a whole new era of cancer research based on the discovery that the failure of cells to die when they should is the reason they become cancerous.

"We really didn't understand how cancer worked. But now we think we do because we're beginning to dissect the molecular basis of cancer," says Dr. Gary K. Schwartz, a medical oncologist at the Memorial Sloan-Kettering Cancer Center.

Dr. Francis S. Collins, director of the federal government's Human Genome Research Institute, agrees. According to Collins, who is overseeing the Human Genome Project, the massive effort to discover all of the approximately 75,000 human genes, "We're heading for a paradigm shift where we will be putting into the clinic magic bullets against cancer that are going to be developed from the glorious outpouring of information that's coming out of basic science research. I believe it probably will happen over the next couple of decades, which means it might be next year or it might be 20 years from now. It won't be longer than that."

For some cancer patients, these magic bullets are already here. Jane, a 57-year-old lab technician from Indiana, thought she was going to die of breast cancer. The cancer had been diagnosed four years earlier and Jane had undergone the standard therapy—a lumpectomy to remove the tumor and chemotherapy to mop up any cancerous cells left behind. For two years she was fine, but then the cancer came back aggressively; it grew rapidly and no amount of chemotherapy could derail it. When open sores appeared on her chest, Jane was sure she had lost the battle.

But death was not in the cards for Jane. She was lucky: she managed to enroll in a study testing a new breast cancer drug called herceptin.

Herceptin doesn't poison cells as most cancer drugs do; instead, it seems to coax them into committing suicide on their own.

"I knew the drug was working after a couple of weeks," says Jane. "The open sores dried up and scabbed over. By the time I saw the doctor again she was totally amazed."

In Jane's case the cancer disappeared completely, but not all women who receive herceptin are as fortunate. Still, the drug's early promise suggests that medical researchers are finally on the right track to developing anticancer drugs that truly work.

Why do cells, especially the kinds that cause cancer, make mistakes? You'd think that after four billion years of evolution, cells would have gotten good enough not to make any mistakes. But if they didn't make any mistakes we would all be protoplasmic, single-cell amoebas. Mistakes drive evolution—they're ingrained into the process of DNA replication. Cancer is a side effect of evolution for long-lived organisms like us.

But evolution has developed many mechanisms to protect us from cancer, including antioxidants that prevent free radicals from damaging genes, white blood cells that gobble up cancerous cells and cell suicide that eliminates potentially harmful cells before they can cause injury. Even though cancer is a threat to us from birth, these powerful defenses keep us cancer-free for most of our lives, or until they, too, succumb to free radical injury.

**In order for cancer to finally gain a footing in the body, a cell's suicide genes need to be knocked out. Free of the body's house-cleaning mandate, damaged cells become slums, attracting all sorts of unsavory characters. Inside these squalid cells, the dangerous new lodgers are genes that become mutated from excessive exposure to free radicals. Many of these slum-dwelling genetic errors simply clutter up the nucleus of the cell—but others can trigger unbridled cell multiplication, the testy hallmark of cancer.**

"The failure of cells to die when they should is the fundamental cause of cancer," asserts geneticist Robert Horvitz. Horvitz was the first to discover normal genes that cause cells to commit suicide, a finding that led to the detection of genes that perform the opposite function—keeping cells alive. One of these human anti-death genes, called bcl-2, can cause cancer when it is mutated. "All you have to do is have bcl-2 be overly active, allowing cells to live much longer than they normally would. These cells may not have suffered any other genetic damage at all but they can be harmed later because they are resistant to programmed cell death and exposed to excessive DNA injury. This can lead to cancer."

The death-defying cells become invincible renegades bent on satisfying their own selfish desire to divide and grow at the expense of their host. Mocking gene-ordered death from within and brushing off the attacks of anticancer drugs and radiation from without, a tumor cell continues to multiply, choking out healthy cells and sucking the life forces from the body. This new knowledge is helping scientists understand why resistant cancers thumb their noses at traditional poison and burn therapies. They had assumed that drugs and radiation kill cancer cells through some form of blunt trauma that causes the cells to blow up. They now understand that these treatments rely on triggering programmed cell death to destroy tumors. When cells refuse to die when they should, the therapies become toothless tigers.

"Everybody asks me why we haven't found a cure for cancer," says Kristin Eckert, a cancer researcher at Pennsylvania State University. "I tell them we're just now finding out all these new things about cancer. I think we're finally on the right track in terms of understanding cancer and coming up with ways of treating it."

The rethinking of cancer dramatically changes its outlook. By finding strategies to reactivate the cell-suicide mechanism, scientists are putting new cancer cures on the horizon. So compelling, in fact, is the promise of chemicals that induce cell suicide that they have been given a name—selective apoptotic anti-neoplastic drugs, or SAANDS. In various ways they are intended to break a cancer cell's stranglehold on immortality and mercifully allow it to die. SAANDS do not trigger apoptosis in normal cells. One of these drugs, Exisulind, is showing promise in men with advanced prostate cancer and is shrinking polyps in people who are susceptible to colon cancer.

Drs. Gary H. Gibbons of Harvard and Burkhard Jansen of the University Hospital, Vienna, restored the suicide mechanism to cancer cells by unlocking the chemical grip of the bcl-2 gene, which had prevented the cells from dying. Cancers disappeared completely in half the animals that had their bcl-2 activity stopped and were then treated with the anticancer drug dacarbazine. The drug was useless against cancers in animals whose bcl-2 activity continued unimpeded.

The bcl-2 gene is helping to explain the mystery of why black males have the highest rate of prostate cancer in the world: they appear to have an altered form of the bcl-2 gene that makes cancer cells much more resistant to suicide. As a result, black males are more prone to prostate cancer and, when they get it, it's a more aggressive form. The mutated bcl-2 gene enables cancer cells to flourish when they would normally die, and it increases the likelihood that the cancer will spread to other parts of the body. (Prostate cancer is diagnosed in more than 300,000 American males each year, but the cure rate is higher than 90 percent when detected early.)

Only two decades ago, many scientists thought they would never understand cancer. Their forlorn assessment was that cancer was too complex, that it probably involved more than 100 different diseases. The era of molecular biology that arose in the 80s gave them the ability to study genes and uncover the secondary cause of cancer: mutated genes—usually DNA that has been blistered by free radicals—that derange critical cell functions and provoke unregulated cell division. Even more important, they have now discovered the fundamental cause of cancer—the failure of damaged cells to die when they are supposed to. By failing to heed their suicide genes, cells give cancer a home.

The message is clear and hopeful: most cancers are preventable. A massive study of more than 44,000 pairs of identical twins, who have identical genes, and fraternal twins, who share about half of the same genes, showed that what the twins ate and how they lived accounted for two-thirds of their cancers. An identical twin who smoked, ate a high-fat diet and didn't exercise was prone to cancer while his or her identical sibling who did not have these risk factors was protected from cancer. Free radicals from a dangerous lifestyle were mutating normal genes and causing cancer in one twin and not in the other. Inherited cancer genes were involved in only one-third of the cancers, mostly as agents that increased the likelihood that the twins would be more vulnerable to free radical damage.

Evolution's most potent defenders against cancer are versatile housekeeping genes such as P-53. Every cell has a copy. P-53 works like a cleaning service, handyman and garbage disposal all in one. The protein made from P-53 has two essential jobs—stopping cell division until damaged DNA can be repaired and activating the suicide pathway if genetic mistakes are too severe to be fixed. The majority of all human cancers involve a P-53 gene that has been either mutated by free radicals or, far less frequently, inherited as a genetic defect. A flawed P-53 gene can no longer pull the switch for cell death.

A healthy P-53 gene is normally a cell's last-ditch self-destruct button. If a cell recognizes that it's going to become cancerous, it turns on the P-53 gene and commits hara-kiri. If you mutate P-53, you deprive the cell of even that last refuge. When it's healthy and working as it should, P-53 neatly eliminates a cell. Like a terminator given instructions to destroy an evil factory, a healthy P-53 suicide gene unleashes proteins that generate a blast of free radicals from a cell's energy producers, mitochondria. In this internal explosion, the free radicals annihilate all of the cell's machinery, from its DNA to its protein building blocks. Riddled to pieces, the shattered cell attracts immune cells, which engulf the debris, leaving no trace.

Researchers are treating many of these P-53-related cancers by giving patients healthy copies of the gene. Encapsulated in a harmless cold virus, thousands of the normal P-53 genes are injected into cancer sites. (Minus its own genes, the virus shell is able to slip into cancer cells without causing infection.) Once delivered to the cancer cells, the good P-53 genes give them a mandate: kill yourselves. Because so many human cancers involve a mutated P-53 gene, the therapy shows promise for treating a wide range of killer cancers, including those that attack the liver, bladder, brain, breast and colon. The approach seems to be working in early tests with lung cancer patients.

Around the world, several hundred patients with advanced cancers have received P-53 gene therapy. In some cases, the cancers have stopped growing and even regressed. Carol, a 58-year-old former secretary from Huntington Beach, California, received infusions of P-53 at UCLA. The treatment caused her ovarian cancer cells to die. "I felt at the edge of death," she says. "If I hadn't enrolled in the study, I wouldn't have been around to see my youngest daughter graduate from pharmacy school." Before the treatment, Carol had to be helped in and out of a car. Now she takes long walks on the beach with her husband.

The P-53 gene may be a good candidate for a cancer vaccine. Proteins made by mutated P-53 genes are bent out of shape and accumulate in cancer cells, unlike the proteins made by normal P-53 genes, which are rapidly excreted from cells. Studies in mice show that immunizing them against the abnormal P-53 protein product protects them from cancer.

In their search for drugs that reactivate apoptosis, scientists were surprised to find that some seemingly simple compounds such as aspirin can trigger cell death in precancerous cells. Regular aspirin users, for instance, have half the rate of colon cancer of nonusers and they also have lower rates of cancers of the esophagus, breast and lung.

Colon cancer is a typical example of how resistance to cell death can eventually turn into cancer and how something like aspirin and other anti-inflammatory agents can prevent it. The first step toward colon cancer is the development of mutations in the suicide genes inside cells in the epithelial lining of the colon. Instead of being routinely sloughed off in about a week, the mutated epithelial cells stay around for many years. Dr. Raymond N. DuBois Jr., a Vanderbilt University cell biologist, found that an enzyme called cox-2 prevents the cells from dying. The enzyme is present in 85 percent of colon cancer cells but not in healthy colon cells. Colon cancer takes a long time to develop, about 10 years. Cells that refuse to die don't proliferate any faster than healthy cells do, but because they don't die, they accumulate. Over time, they slowly form masses of tissue that bulge out from the intestinal lining like mushrooms.

Since these bulbous masses, or polyps, stay around so much longer than they should, they become growing targets for random free-radical hits. The odds are greatly increased that a growth-regulating gene inside a polyp cell will get hit by a free radical or other cancer-inducing substance and become mutated. Once mutated, the gene sends out signals for the cell to divide rapidly. Free of its commitment to kill itself and with fresh instructions to multiply, the cell turns cancerous.

When DuBois knocked out the cox-2 enzyme with genetic-engineering wizardry, the colon cancer cells withered and died. Aspirin, it turned out, did the same thing: when DuBois exposed death-resistant colon cells to aspirin, the aspirin combined with the anti-death enzyme and blocked its activity, causing the polyp-forming cells to deflate and perish.

Doctors are hopeful that anti-inflammatory medications can help prevent colon cancer in people who have an inherited disorder called familial polyposis, which is characterized by the growth of enormous numbers of colon polyps that can become cancerous. When they take an anti-inflammatory drug called Sulindac, their polyps regress. When they stop taking the drug, the polyps start growing again.

Dr. Edward Giovannucci of the Harvard Medical School and Brigham and Women's Hospital in Boston, who heads the Nurses Health Study of more than 120,000 American nurses, found that the nurses who took aspirin frequently for 20 years or more had a 44 percent lower risk of colorectal cancer than those who did not take aspirin. "I think that aspirin and these other anti-inflammatory agents work at the very earliest stage, preventing the polyps from progressing and becoming malignant," he says.

Taking aspirin is a simple and inexpensive way to prevent colon cancer. And some doctors are now recommending that people at risk for colorectal cancer take a single aspirin tablet (325 milligrams) every other day. (A similar dose of aspirin has already been linked to a significantly lower risk of heart attack.)

The long-standing nurses study also reveals that women who take estrogen supplements after menopause for at least five years can reduce their risk of cancer of the colon and rectum by 35 percent. How estrogen reduces this risk is not yet clear, but the hormone appears to exert a calming effect on cells that line the colon and rectum, probably by reducing free radical activity. This protection fades when women stop taking estrogen.

Women at high risk of breast cancer are turning to a drug called tamoxifen, the first medication shown to prevent breast cancer. The hormonal medication—which has already been used successfully to prevent the recurrence of breast cancer in women who have undergone surgery, radiation or chemotherapy—can cut nearly in half the risk of breast cancer in women who don't have the disease but are at high risk of developing it. Many types of breast cancer are sensitive to estrogen, which stimulates their growth. Tamoxifen blocks estrogen receptors on breast cancer cells, which prevents the hormone from activating cell division. Excessive cell division increases the rate of genetic damage from free radicals. Tamoxifen slightly raises the risk of uterine cancer, but its benefits in preventing breast cancer in high-risk women outweigh this drawback because uterine cancer is relatively easy to diagnose at an early stage and cure.

A drug similar to tamoxifen, called raloxifene, may provide even more benefits than tamoxifen with fewer side effects. Raloxifene is a synthetic version of estrogen. It prevents osteoporosis as estrogen does and it may reduce the risk of breast cancer by up to 70 percent. The drug also may decrease the risk of heart disease, another of estrogen's benefits. But unlike estrogen, raloxifene does not appear to increase the risk of uterine cancer;

raloxifene binds to breast cell estrogen receptors but does not stimulate the cells to divide.

Scientists have discovered some even simpler ways to prevent cancer. Antioxidants, especially those found in fruits and vegetables, can block the free radical damage to DNA that can lead to cancer. People who eat the most fruits and vegetables have half the cancer rate of people who eat the least amounts of these foods. That this is true can easily be observed in your friends, family members and acquaintances who are healthy. What are they eating? Probably plenty of vegetables, fruits, whole grains and legumes and very little high-fat meat, cheese, fast foods and snacks.

"I eat lots of vegetables because I like them," says Richard, a 62-year-old San Francisco journalist. Richard's lunch is usually a bowl of bean or vegetable soup and a luncheon salad. "We're supposed to eat at least five servings of vegetables and fruits a day. Since one serving is half a cup, I figure my big lunch salad is equal to about five servings." With fruit for breakfast and more vegetables at dinner, Richard is among the smart people who consume more than 10 servings of these foods a day, almost eliminating their chances of getting cancer.

Based on promising dietary studies, a number of trials are under way to test the ability of individual antioxidants to prevent cancer. For some antioxidants, the study results have been mixed, but they have led to a more sophisticated understanding of the beneficial molecules.

Lycopene, a member of the vitamin A family and an antioxidant that gives tomatoes their red color, has already been linked to a 45-percent reduction in prostate cancer among men who eat at least 10 servings a week of tomato-based foods. In addition, lycopene substantially reduces the risk of cancers of the lung and stomach and is helpful in preventing cancers of the breast, colon, rectum, pancreas, cervix, esophagus and mouth.

Low levels of the B vitamin folic acid (or folate) are linked to an increase in genetic mutations from free radicals and a decline in the ability of cells to repair DNA damage—major risk factors for cancer. Both can be reversed with adequate intake of folate. The national decline in colon cancer cases appears to be the result of increased consumption of folate by Americans since 1973, when manufacturers began fortifying cereals with the vitamin and adding it to multivitamin supplements.

The beta carotene story remains a puzzle because the compound, a precursor of vitamin A, seems to act in contradictory ways. Beta carotene can act as a pro-oxidant, which induces the production of free radicals (especially in smokers), as well as an antioxidant. In one study, researchers found that lung cancer among smokers given beta carotene increased by 28 percent while lung cancers decreased by 20 percent among former smokers who took the same antioxidant.

"This raises the possibility that former smokers are responding favorably to beta carotene and it certainly raises an even stronger possibility that they are responding differently than current smokers," says Dr. Gilbert Omenn of the University of Michigan, who headed the study.

Similar puzzling results were reported in an earlier study in which heavy smokers were given beta carotene and vitamin E. Beta carotene was linked to an increase in lung cancer, while vitamin E was found to decrease the rate of prostate cancer. One preliminary conclusion from these studies is that antioxidants seem to work to prevent the genetic damage that induces cancer, but once cells have become cancerous, it may be too late for some antioxidants to reverse the process. For people who continue to smoke, free radicals overwhelm their antioxidant defenses. Another lesson is that antioxidants work best when taken together.

Selenium was once considered a relatively weak antioxidant, but it builds an amazing wall of protection against cancer. Selenium is an essential mineral that is used for making glutathione peroxidase, a potent enzyme that the body uses to snuff out free radicals. In addition to acting on its own as a free-radical neutralizer, selenium gives comfort and strength to other antioxidants, including vitamin E.

The discovery of selenium's healing powers came as a surprise to scientists because the mineral had failed to reduce the rate of skin cancer in an earlier study. When the researchers reviewed the data more carefully, however, they found that the study volunteers who took selenium had 50 percent fewer deaths from all types of cancer. Although selenium did not have much effect on harmless skin cancers, it seemed to be a potent force against killer cancers. Prostate cancer showed the biggest decline—63 percent. Vegetables and grains are rich in selenium, as are fish, shellfish, meat, egg yolks, garlic and Brazil nuts. Many doctors are recommending that people take selenium supplements to make sure they are getting an adequate amount.

The selenium story illustrates once again the crucial balance between antioxidants and free radicals and how cancer and other diseases can result when the balance tips in favor of free radicals. If you have low levels of antioxidants such as selenium and your fat consumption is high, your risk of cancer is increased dramatically. By contrast, a high intake of antioxidants and a low intake of fat significantly decrease your cancer risk. Fat consumption and cancer have a deadly association. Men who eat the most animal fat increase their risk of developing prostate cancer by 75 to 130 percent. Joe used to enjoy high-fat foods—and he paid the price with a cancerous prostate that threatened to kill him. But he was able to reverse the cancer by drastically cutting back on the fat in his diet.

Sloan-Kettering's Dr. Fair first noticed the favorable effect of diet when Joe and several other patients whose late-stage prostate cancers were resistant to standard treatments went on highly restricted diets. Like Joe, they had asked in desperation if they could go on special diets because they had heard that doing so might help fight their cancer. The diets varied—macrobiotic, vegetarian or rice—but they all had one thing in common: they were very low in fat. Any diet that limited fat to 20 percent or less of total calories produced a remarkable decline in the blood level of a protein called Prostate Specific Antigen (PSA), which is used to diagnose and evaluate prostate cancer. Numbers dropped from high levels in the 20s and 30s, indicating dangerous cancer activity, to as low as 0.4 to 2.5, indicating the tumors were dormant.

"My goal is to be able to tell a 60-year-old man with prostate cancer that he can do something to slow the growth of the tumor so it won't impact his life span for 30 years. If we can slow the growth of prostate cancer, which already is a slow-growing tumor, that would be tantamount to a cure for men who are in their 60s and 70s," Fair says.

The studies of these relatively simple measures—eating a low-fat or high-fiber diet or taking compounds such as vitamins, aspirin and estrogen—are especially important because they show that people can do things to prevent cancer even late in life.

Although we are witnessing incredible advances in understanding cancer and developing promising treatments, it remains a cagey adversary. Cancer has found a way to subvert every defense the body has evolved against it—even using one defense against another. Such is the case with telomeres, DNA caps at the ends of chromosomes that are designed to prevent a cell from dividing in an uncontrolled fashion. Every time a cell divides, a bit of the telomere tip is nicked off. When telomeres are reduced to stubs, after about 50 divisions, a cell stops dividing and becomes senescent or commits suicide. DNA is most susceptible to free-radical mutations when cells are dividing. By shutting down cell division, telomere shortening serves as an anti-cancer defense.

However, some cancers, such as those of the testicle and bone marrow, have outwitted this protective mechanism by turning on a gene that makes telomerase, an enzyme that rebuilds telomere tips, thereby enabling a cell to go on dividing. In most cells, the telomerase gene is supposed to be shut off and turned on only when it is needed during normal cell division, which occurs regularly in the liver and in the lining of the intestine and during scar formation. Turning telomerase on permanently could have grave consequences: cells that continue to divide way beyond their normal limit run the risk of incurring free radical damage to their genes, which can lead to cancer.

In the unfolding new understanding of cancer, scientists are beginning to recognize that some viruses can cause cancer by hijacking the genes that regulate cell suicide. Unable to die as they normally would, the hijacked cells slowly grow, providing a safe haven for the virus and exposing the genes in the cells to more free radical damage. For example, the human papillomavirus (HPV), which causes genital warts, is the major cause of cervical cancer in women. The warts are made of cells that the virus has prevented from dying. Living well beyond their allotted time, the cells become targets of free radical damage, increasing their chances of becoming cancerous.

The new knowledge of cancer is replacing decades of hopelessness with a sense of optimism. "We've made great strides in identifying the mutated genes that cause cancer and figuring out what has to be corrected," says molecular virologist Nancy Raab-Traub of the University of North Carolina at Chapel Hill. "I used to think I wouldn't see any cancer cures in my lifetime, but now I do see them—actual genetic cures."

# 5

# *Preventing Heart Disease*

Of all the diseases that strike humans, from cancer to AIDS, the one that kills the most Americans is man-made. Heart disease, the No. 1 killer of both men and women, and its deadly sidekick, stroke, the No. 3 killer, are unnatural causes of death.

Of the 5.7 billion people on earth, four billion don't get heart attacks or strokes because they live the kind of life that evolution prepared the human body for—engaging in physical activity and eating a diet low in fat and high in vegetables, fruits and whole grains. People in modern societies have adopted dangerous new lifestyles—smoking, overeating and being sedentary—with which their bodies don't know how to cope. Heart disease is an over-reaction to these drastically changing lifestyles. Three out of four Americans are overweight and one out of three is obese.

New research is on the verge of knocking heart disease off the list of the top 10 killers. "We can eliminate most of the heart disease and stroke in this country simply by applying current knowledge, even if we don't learn anything more," insists Mier J. Stampfer, professor of epidemiology and nutrition at the Harvard School of Public Health. "We're already seeing that happen among people with better education who are taking advantage of the new information. Heart disease is not nearly as common among educated people as it was several decades ago."

Fundamentally, the human body likes to be treated like a finely-tuned racing machine. But more and more, we are treating our bodies like jalopies and they are clogging up and breaking down on us. The body has learned how to fight an infinite variety of infectious germs and devised ways to cleanse itself of cancer. It can fix broken genes and repair damaged tissue and it knows how to marshal its resources when food is scarce. What the body has never learned to do, however, is to handle a constant overload of fat in the blood.

In the bloodstream, fat is ferried around by proteins called lipoproteins. Low-density lipoproteins (LDLs) deliver cholesterol to cells for building membranes and making hormones. High-density lipoproteins (HDLs) remove excess cholesterol from the blood. This delicate balance between LDLs and HDLs can be upset by a high-fat diet, which creates more fat-laden LDLs than the body knows what to do with. Like butter that sits out too long, fat-laden LDLs can turn rancid from free radical damage.

When this occurs, the body becomes confused. Mighty macrophages, the immune system's white blood cells that attack and eliminate germs and other potentially harmful invaders, are overwhelmed. They have no problem gobbling up and getting rid of a handful of spoiled cholesterol particles in the blood, but faced with a regular torrent of rancid LDLs, they lose control. Like drunks who stumble into a vat of wine and find that the only way out is to drink the vat dry, the macrophages swallow more and more of the spoiled cholesterol particles. Engorged with fat, the macrophages squeeze in among the cells that line arteries and hide there. Still gobbling up cholesterol, they grow to enormous size, transforming themselves into sodden foam cells. Alarmed at their blundering, the immune system rallies to the site. But it, too, becomes confused; its weapons are defenseless against the bloated macrophages that it recognizes as parts of "self"—not enemies.

The immune system makes matters worse. It fires its weapons, but instead of striking a foe, they hit their own ammunition dump, causing an inflammatory explosion that calls in even more macrophages. But they also take part in the fat feast. Smooth muscle cells from inside the artery lining are ordered to the front line in a misguided effort to repair damage that doesn't need repair. Not knowing what else to do, the muscle cells engulf fat particles and grow bigger and bigger until they also turn into insatiable foam cells. At the same time, inflammation worsens the problem by mass-producing free radicals.

As the over-stuffed products of this errant response build up, fatty streaks of foam cells start to appear in the artery lining, heralding the beginning of heart disease. Over time, the fatty streaks thicken into deposits called plaques, which narrow the arteries. This process is called atherosclerosis, or, more descriptively, hardening of the arteries. The stage is now set for a heart attack or stroke: the plaque can rupture or a blood clot can form, either of which can block the narrowed vessel, shutting off the blood supply to the heart or brain.

The fact that only a small percentage of the world's population dies in this way has become so evident that medical researchers now believe that the killers of the heart and brain can be completely disarmed. "Coronary artery disease is not part of human nature or of the aging process," says Dr. Edgar Haber, director of the Harvard School of Public Health's Center for the Prevention of Cardiovascular Disease. "It does not exist in many groups outside of developed and developing countries and, ultimately, should be fully preventable."

How quickly heart disease can be prevented was demonstrated by a remarkable turn of events that occurred in Poland after the fall of communism. Under the 30-year rule of communism, during which the government provided meat, dairy products and other high-fat food subsidies to all citizens, deaths from heart attacks doubled. When the food subsidies stopped after the government collapsed, people in Poland were forced to decrease their consumption of meat and butter and increase their consumption of vegetables and fruits. In four short years, starting in 1991, Poland experienced the fastest and biggest drop in heart attack deaths ever recorded—a 25-percent plunge. Stroke deaths declined 10 percent.

The medical assault on heart disease began in 1948 with the start of the famous Framingham Heart Study. By carefully assessing the eating, exercise and other lifestyle habits of every resident of the small town of Framingham, Massachusetts, researchers began to discover the risk factors for heart disease—elevated cholesterol, cigarette smoking and high blood pressure. The landmark study continues to uncover new heart risks, such as the importance of the relative proportions in the blood of HDL and LDL.

The Framingham study has also identified factors that protect people against clogged arteries. Its most recent finding: for every increase of three servings of fruits and vegetables a day, stroke risk decreases 20 percent. Earlier findings showed similar protection for the heart.

"The bottom line in the Framingham study is that you can go into any town in the world and, with a few simple tests, identify all the people who are going to have a heart attack or stroke," says Dr. William P. Castelli, the long-time medical director of the study. "We never treated anyone in the Framingham study. But now I'm on the other side. I'm aggressively managing all of their risk factors to give them a shot at missing these diseases completely."

The realization that a person can avoid a heart attack or stroke by reducing or eliminating his or her risk factors began to emerge in the mid 1960s when heart attack deaths were at an all-time high, about 240 deaths per 100,000 people annually. Then, to the amazement of medical researchers, heart attack deaths began a precipitous decline. Today they are about half the rate they were nearly four decades ago, but the numbers are still huge—one and a half million heart attacks annually and 500,000 deaths. Strokes have undergone an even steeper decline, falling about 65 percent since the early 1960s when stroke deaths stood at about 80 per 100,000 people. Nevertheless, they remain unacceptably high at 700,000 strokes a year and 150,000 deaths.

Why did the rate of heart attack and stroke deaths fall so suddenly? Certainly better medical care played a role, but lifestyle changes appear to have been far more important. The dramatic drop in mortality followed the first messages from public health officials warning of the dangers of high cholesterol and cigarettes. And starting in the 1950s, fresh fruits and vegetables became available throughout the country year-round, providing increasing numbers of people with vitamins and the thousands of other antioxidant compounds found in these plants.

**Although scientists were able to identify the major risk factors for both heart disease and stroke—cigarette smoking, high cholesterol levels, high blood pressure, diabetes, physical inactivity and obesity—they didn't know how they all fit together to produce disease. With the aid of biology's new ability to probe individual molecules, researchers are now beginning to discover the underlying cause of heart disease and stroke—free radical damage—and learn how to prevent it, sometimes with simple measures.**

"For so long, we've been thinking that heart disease was just a problem of too much saturated fat and cholesterol," says nutrition expert Walter Willet of the Harvard School of Public Health. "The balance between antioxidants and free radical damage is turning out to be important. The picture that's emerging is that inadequate protective factors—particularly antioxidants, fiber and folic acid—are going to be more important in the long run."

Harvard's pioneering studies of thousands of doctors and nurses showed that people who eat diets rich in fruits and vegetables have the lowest death rates from heart attack and stroke. The doctors study also showed that men who eat 25 to 30 grams of fiber each day have a 35 percent reduced risk of heart disease compared with men who eat 10 to 15 grams of fiber. A person who eats more than eight servings of fruits and vegetables a day reduces his or her risk of having a stroke by 60 percent compared with a person who eats fewer than two servings.

All over the world, heart disease and stroke are rare among people who eat lots of fruits and vegetables. Antioxidants can even be bottled. Red wine contains large amounts of antioxidants from grapes, a discovery that helps to explain the French paradox—the low rate of heart disease among the French despite their high-fat diet. Their tradition of drinking red wine with meals appears to offset the effects of the free radicals from the fat.

Eating 10 or more servings of fruits and vegetables a day pumps so many antioxidants into our bodies that they can be measured in our breath. Such a massive dose of antioxidants flushes out free radicals and cleanses our arteries. Our blood flows clear; cholesterol particles, undamaged by free radicals, glide smoothly, posing no threat of heart disease.

How do the scores of known and unknown antioxidants in fruits and vegetables provide such a strong defense against free radical damage? Johns Hopkins University researchers, headed by Dr. Edgar R. Miller, wanted to find an answer to this question. Of concern was the destruction that free radicals do to LDL particles. In their study, one group of men ate a diet low in fruits and vegetables (only about four servings a day) and high in fat (with 37 percent of calories coming from fat). A second group ate nine servings of fruits and vegetables daily along with a high-fat diet. A third group ate about 10 servings of fruits and vegetables a day and a low-fat diet. To find out how well the men's bodies were neutralizing free radicals in the bloodstream, the scientists measured the amount of a gas, ethane, in the men's breath. Ethane is released from the lungs as part of the wreckage that results when free radicals bombard LDL cholesterol, providing vivid evidence of free radical damage.

The men in the study who ate the high-fat, low-vegetable-and-fruit diet were churning out free radicals at a dangerous pace, their breath clouded with ethane. The men who ate nine servings of fruits and vegetables along with fatty foods fared better, but their ethane level was still in the danger zone. The men who ate lots of fruits and vegetables and little fat were the luckiest of all—their breath emitted almost no ethane. Carotenoids, flavonoids, tocopherols, lutein, vitamins E and C and other antioxidants in their 10 daily servings of fruits and vegetables were squelching free radicals before they could cause harm.

Scientists recently discovered one of the most powerful plant antioxidants, lycopene, which is most plentiful in tomatoes but is also present in pink grapefruit and watermelon. Like a molecular blotter, lycopene circulates in the blood and sops up free radicals that could otherwise damage

LDL and start the build-up of fatty deposits in arteries. Cooking tomatoes frees lycopene from cell walls, making more of the antioxidant available for the body to absorb. Tomato sauce, for example, has four times more absorbable lycopene than fresh tomatoes. A major study has shown that men who eat the most tomato-based products—including ketchup, tomato paste and tomato juice—have half the risk of developing heart disease of men who consume the least amount of lycopene-rich foods.

The tasty and popular Mediterranean diet—which contains a small amount of meat and lots of vegetables, fruits, legumes and cereals and some fish, low-fat cheese and olive oil and other vegetable oils—has been known to protect against heart disease. Enjoyed by millions of people in Italy, Greece and other countries around the sun-splashed Mediterranean Sea, the diet has spread throughout the world. People who consume the abundant harvests of the land and sea have one of the lowest rates of heart disease in the world. They are protected by nature's bounty, including such potent lifesavers as antioxidants in vegetables and fruits and cholesterol-lowering oils in olives, nuts, seeds and fish. The alphalinolenic acid found in olives and nuts and omega-3 fatty acid found in fish act as antioxidants in the lining of arteries by preventing inflammation, which generates free radicals. They also can calm potentially deadly irregular heart rhythms and reduce the formation of blood clots. People who eat fish at least twice a week, especially oily fish such as salmon, have a 50 to 70 percent lower risk of having a fatal heart attack.

It's as if nature, in its wisdom, created a pharmacopoeia for health made out of tasty and nutritious foods that have been around for thousands of years but out of reach until modern transportation made them ubiquitous. Yet it is only now that we are recognizing the potency of these natural healers to actually treat heart disease. Dr. Michel de Lorgeril of Lyon, France, divided 400 heart attack victims into two groups and asked one group to eat a Mediterranean diet and the other to eat their regular Western diet. After four years, those who were eating the Mediterranean diet had one-third to one-half the risk of having a second heart attack of those consuming their customary fare.

One of the major discoveries to come out of the Framingham and Harvard studies is that a high cholesterol level is not the major cause of heart disease, as once was thought. Most people with heart disease have so-called normal cholesterol levels. Three other culprits have emerged as independent precursors to heart disease and stroke:

*    Insulin resistance—the first step on the road to adult-onset, or type 2, diabetes—which doubles the risk of heart disease
*    A deficiency in the B-complex vitamins—folic acid, B-6 and B-12—which also doubles the risk of heart disease
*    Long-standing, low-grade infection in the arteries, which triples the risk of heart attack and doubles the risk of stroke.

These risk factors for heart disease appear to use some of the same biological mechanisms to produce their damage—and the free radical is the thread that links them. In a person with insulin resistance, insulin levels increase in the blood, disrupting a number of biological functions. One of the most damaging changes occurs in the LDL molecule. LDL does not increase, as it does from eating a high-fat diet, but it undergoes a deadly transformation—it becomes small and dense and more susceptible to free radical damage. Being overweight is the primary cause of elevated insulin levels, so losing excess weight may lower the risk of heart disease from insulin resistance.

Low levels of the B-vitamins folic acid and vitamins B-6 and B-12 increase the risk of heart disease by causing a dangerous rise in the blood of a chemical called homocysteine. A person can have a normal cholesterol count, but if his or her homocysteine level is high, he or she is in danger of heart disease from excessive free radical production. Homocysteine causes trouble in many different ways, mostly by generating huge quantities of free radicals, primarily superoxide and hydrogen peroxide. These destructive sparks damage artery walls and LDL and promote the formation of blood clots, all of which greatly increase the risk of heart attack and stroke.

Homocysteine is so dangerous that it is now listed as a risk factor for heart disease on a par with smoking and a high cholesterol level. A homocysteine level just 12 percent above normal increases a person's risk of heart attack by 200 percent. Taking at least 400 micrograms of folic acid daily, along with vitamins B6 and B12, reduces homocysteine to normal levels, significantly lowering the risk of heart disease. (Elevated homocysteine levels have also been linked to cancers of the breast, ovary and pancreas.)

The long-term Harvard nurses study found that women with the highest levels of folic acid and vitamin B-6 had half the risk of heart disease of women with the lowest levels. The women in the study got most of their folic acid and vitamin B-6 from multivitamin supplements and fortified cold cereals. Foods that are naturally rich in folate include green, leafy vegetables; orange juice; eggs; and broccoli. Good sources of vitamin B-6 include bananas, chicken, beef, potatoes, fish and whole grains. University of Washington researchers estimate that one out of 10 heart attack deaths, a total of 56,000 each year, could be prevented simply by increasing the intake of folic acid and the other B vitamins—through diet or vitamin supplements—to reduce homocysteine levels.

The ability of folic acid and vitamin B-6 to reduce homocysteine levels in the blood may be responsible for the bulk of the protection against heart disease found in the nurses study. The strongest protection against heart disease is achieved with 400 micrograms a day of folic acid and 3 milligrams a day of vitamin B-6. Both these amounts are considerably above the RDAs of 180 micrograms of folic acid per day for women and 200 micrograms for men and 1.6 milligrams of vitamin B-6 per day for women and 2 milligrams for men. As with the RDAs for other nutrients, it appears that the allowances for folic acid and vitamin B-6 are set much too low and that doubling them is necessary for optimum health.

Systemic infection in the arteries causes heart disease by triggering inflammation. The inflammatory response produces an excessive amount of free radicals, which can damage the lining of arteries. Cholesterol that has been damaged by free radicals has an easier time entering the artery lining, which can initiate the plaque-building process even when cholesterol levels are normal. Inflammation leaves a chemical byproduct in the blood called plasma C-reactive protein. Men with the highest levels of C-reactive protein in their blood have a threefold increased risk of heart attack and twice the risk of stroke. Above-normal levels of the protein can predict a person's risk of having a first heart attack six to eight years in the future. Once tests are developed to easily detect C-reactive protein, people will gain sufficient forewarning of a heart attack to head it off with prevention strategies.

The Harvard researchers who pinpointed the link between infection and heart disease also found that aspirin can prevent heart trouble. Scientists originally thought that aspirin blocked heart disease primarily by preventing the formation of blood clots, which can clog arteries. But aspirin (and possibly other anti-inflammatory agents) may also prevent heart disease by curbing inflammation in the arteries. No one has seen this more clearly than biochemist Balz Frei, director of the Linus Pauling Institute at Oregon State University, whose experiments documented the insidious process by which free radicals from cigarette smoke damage cholesterol.

Two of the best-known antioxidants, vitamins C and E, work in different ways to protect LDL particles from the ravages of free radicals. Vitamin C, which is water soluble, is active in the bloodstream and serves as the first line of defense against free radicals in cigarette smoke. Vitamin E, which is fat soluble, is the second line of defense, manning battlements in the membranes of LDL particles and protecting them from free radical damage.

In test-tube experiments, Frei exposed plasma (blood stripped of its red and white cells) from human volunteers to cigarette smoke. The plasma contained natural amounts of vitamins C and E that had entered the blood from fruits and vegetables they had eaten. Plasma also contains LDL particles. When the plasma was exposed to cigarette smoke, vitamin C in the plasma attacked the free radicals in the smoke and neutralized them. The vitamin provided this strong defense with great efficiency until its supply in the blood ran out. When vitamin C was depleted, free radicals started attacking the cholesterol. At first they were kept at bay by vitamin E in the LDL membrane. But as vitamin E was used up, the cholesterol became vulnerable to damage from free radicals.

Frei found that adding new supplies of vitamins C and E to the plasma could prevent this damage. "You need to replenish vitamins E and C all the time," he says. "That's why we have to take them up in our diet. We can never really stop doing that."

Vitamin C can also benefit people who already have heart disease. Consuming 500 milligrams of vitamin C daily improves blood vessel function in people with heart disease, prevents the chest pains of angina and reduces the risk of heart attack and stroke. Circulating in the blood, vitamin C prevents free radical damage to nitric oxide, a compound the body uses to relax blood vessels, inhibit the formation of blood clots and reduce the risk of plaque rupture.

Since vitamin E is a last line of defense, scientists are trying to figure out how much is needed to provide protection against free radical injury. In studies with human volunteers, Dr. Ishwarlal Jialal of the University of Texas Southwestern Medical Center has found that taking 400 IUs or more of vitamin E daily provides the best protection against LDL injury. The RDA for vitamin E is only a fraction of that—15 IUs. "This amount may be reasonable for preventing vitamin-E-deficiency disorders, but if you want to protect LDLs, you have to go much higher. You need to move into the realm of optimum health," Jialal says.

This creates a problem. Since it is almost impossible to get 400 IUs of vitamin E from your diet, you may need to take pills containing high doses of the vitamin to avoid heart disease. "If this hypothesis is proven, there's no doubt in my mind that the way to go is supplementation with vitamin E," he says.

The same free radical protection conferred by vitamins E and C in the test tube also has been found to work in people. And the vitamins act quickly. Volunteers given 1,000 milligrams of vitamin C and 800 IUs of vitamin E before they ate a high-fat meal were protected against the free radical onslaught created by the fat coursing through their blood. The volunteers who didn't take the vitamins before eating a high-fat meal were not protected; high-resolution ultrasound images revealed that their arteries were under siege and had become stiffer and less flexible. This abnormal activity caused by the clash between free radicals and the linings of arteries lasted four hours. By contrast, the arteries of volunteers who had taken the vitamins in advance of the high-fat meal remained smooth and supple.

Cambridge University researchers in England recently reported the first direct evidence that vitamin E can dramatically reduce the risk of heart attacks in people with severe heart disease. Patients randomly assigned daily doses of either 400 IUs or 800 IUs of vitamin E had only one-fourth the risk of nonfatal heart attacks of patients who received a placebo. This study supplies a crucial missing link that population studies could only hint at. Since the assignment to vitamin E or placebo was random, the benefit can't be explained by anything other than the vitamin itself. Several large-scale studies are under way to determine if vitamin E can prevent heart disease in healthy people.

Vitamin E may also be able to cut the risk of stroke in half, according to results from the four-year Northern Manhattan Stroke Study. Following 850 people, whose average age was 69, the study showed that those who had never had a stroke were twice as likely to be taking vitamin supplements as those who had had strokes.

Using a vitamin to help maintain good health is appealing to a lot of people because it doesn't require much effort or a prescription and it's affordable. Even though vitamins have been around for a long time, scientific understanding about what they can do is still in its infancy. There is no question that people who eat diets rich in vitamins and other antioxidants have the lowest rates of heart disease, but the power of vitamin supplements to do the same has not yet been proven beyond a shadow of a doubt. Why wouldn't doctors want to give everyone vitamin E supplements and reduce the number of heart disease cases by 50 percent? Many would—they're just waiting for the research to prove conclusively that it works.

6

# *Preventing Diabetes: A Modern Epidemic*

At the tender age of 16, Sandra, who has been 25 percent overweight for most of her young life, was recently diagnosed with adult-onset diabetes. She is not alone. An alarming number of children are developing this form of diabetes, called type 2, which previously affected only people in their 50s and 60s.

"It's still hard for me to believe that I have the same disease that some of my older relatives have," says Sandra.

First diagnosed in 1979, type 2 diabetes in children constitutes a frightening new phenomenon. Children used to get only type 1, or juvenile, diabetes, which results from the destruction of insulin-producing cells in the pancreas and comes on rapidly with severe, life-threatening symptoms. By contrast, the adult form develops slowly and stealthily—the result of years of poor health habits.

Today, nearly one out of 3 children with diabetes has the adult type. This dramatic lowering of the age barrier is a consequence of the "domino effect" of two new, tightly interwoven trends—obesity and inactivity—that are driving the head-snapping acceleration of diabetes in grownups and doing the same for children, cruelly marking them for heart disease, blindness, amputations and early death.

The trend is most visible in the growing obesity of Americans and others around the world. In the U.S., one of three Americans is obese and two of three teenagers don't engage in regular vigorous physical activity.

Obesity among children is climbing fast, now reaching adult levels. Type 2 diabetes strikes Americans at the rate of one new case every 52 seconds and threatens to overwhelm developing nations as they switch to Westernized lifestyles that emphasize rich foods and leisure. Since the mid-1980s, the number of global diabetes cases has more than tripled, affecting more than 100 million people. In some Third World countries, diabetes is set to explode.

While an estimated 16 million Americans have type 2 diabetes, only about half have been diagnosed. Unlike infectious diseases, which were the primary cause of death in the U.S. before the 1950s, type 2 diabetes is a lifestyle disease like cancer, heart disease and stroke. Also unlike infections, which are usually painful and visible, lifestyle killers tend to be silent, taking years to do their destruction, prompted by a poor diet, inactivity and harmful behaviors such as smoking.

**The human body did not evolve to take life easy. We have inherited a Stone Age metabolism that is dangerously out of place in the 21st century, where food is ample and convenient. After struggling for millions of years to escape the threat of famine and to make survival easier, humans are learning a cruel lesson about the good life: it's filling our bodies with free radicals and killing us. The energy machine that keeps us moving and thinking is overheating and burning up, producing an excessive and constant shower of free radicals as our risk of developing diabetes greatly increases.**

Type 2 diabetes is a hereditary disease in the sense that genes make a person vulnerable to it and the disorder often occurs in members of the same family. But even if diabetes is common in a family, only the risk of diabetes is passed on to children, not the certainty of developing the disease. The genes become harmful only under stresses such as those caused by being overweight and inactive.

The genetic predisposition to diabetes varies markedly among populations. Western Europeans, who have a long history of food abundance, appear to be somewhat less susceptible to diabetes than people who never have known anything but frugal living. Growing evidence suggests that people in Asia and other developing countries are genetically more likely to get diabetes than people of Western European heritage. Following their traditional diet and frugal way of life, Asians seem to survive relatively free of diabetes. In China, for example, where many people still have a life of frugality and hard physical work, only one percent of the adult population has diabetes. Once Asians adopt Western diets and lifestyles, however, diabetes rates soar: among Chinese immigrants living a modernized life in Mauritius, the diabetes rate is already up to 20 percent of the population.

Indians migrating from Southeast Asia to London have 50 percent more heart disease and diabetes than native British residents, even though the Indians are not as obese as the British and their cholesterol levels are lower. Egypt has become another victim of the diabetes explosion. In 1930, only 10 percent of the adult population had type 2 diabetes; today, 45 percent of adult Egyptians have the disease.

Arizona's Pima Indians are a striking example of how genes and lifestyle can collide. Once lean and healthy when they lived on a grain diet, most have become obese after adopting the high-calorie American diet. Half of the Pimas now have diabetes and, although their overall cholesterol levels are generally normal, deaths from heart attack have skyrocketed. The slow evolution of lifestyle diseases has been much more explosive in communities like the Pima Indians because of their genetic predisposition and the fact that they've never been exposed to this kind of lifestyle before.

Type 2 diabetes strikes when the pancreas, an irregular-shaped gland behind the stomach, becomes a victim of the battle of the bulge—waistline fat. The pancreas fails to produce insulin in amounts necessary for the body to use the sugar glucose efficiently, causing it to build up in the blood and triggering a variety of problems that, untreated, can lead to heart disease, hypertension and cholesterol disorders. Diabetes causes damage in tissues throughout the body because the excess sugar in the blood generates dangerously high levels of free radicals, which scorch cell surface proteins, turning them into a sticky residue like that found on the bottom of a burned pot. This burned residue creates deadening cross-links between proteins, a process called glycosylation.

Glucose levels just slightly higher than normal can cause heart disease. A study of more than 7,000 middle-aged British men, who had no known health problems, found that those who had glucose levels somewhat above normal had a 30 to 40 percent increased risk of developing heart disease. The men were followed for more than nine years. Of the men who developed heart disease, elevated glucose stood out as the probable cause, over traditional risk factors such as smoking, high cholesterol, high blood pressure, obesity and high triglyceride levels.

Glucose is the fuel that runs our brains and all the cells of our bodies: we wouldn't have a thought or a muscle contraction without it. But, like any fuel, glucose can be dangerous. As the body works to meet its energy needs, it is constantly on guard to ensure that glucose is available when needed and that it is hoarded away as fat for future use when food is not available. This energy equilibrium is so delicate that even a slight deviation can be harmful. Too little glucose and a person can quickly go into a coma and die. Too much glucose can lead to an ever-escalating production of free radicals. Like the overheating core of a nuclear reactor, free radicals destroy blood vessels, nerves and other tissues—the body's equivalent of a meltdown.

Scientists and doctors have struggled for years to develop ways to maintain this equilibrium. Insulin, a hormone that enables cells to use glucose, was discovered in the 1920s. Injected daily, it has become a lifesaver for people with type 1 diabetes, who do not produce enough insulin on their own, allowing excess glucose to build up in their blood. Unlike people with type 1 diabetes, people with type 2 diabetes do produce insulin and often a lot of insulin, but it isn't enough to prevent sugar from building up in their blood.

In the 1990s, scientists found that type 1 and type 2 diabetes are only a small part of a much bigger problem when they discovered two other forms of the disease that pose a major threat to health—insulin resistance and impaired glucose tolerance. Together, type 2 diabetes, impaired glucose tolerance and insulin resistance may affect as many as 30 to 45 percent of Americans between the ages of 30 and 65. After 65, the risk is even higher. Insulin resistance is thought to be the most widespread, affecting between 10 and 25 percent of the population. Impaired glucose tolerance, which affects an estimated 20 million Americans, raises sugar in the blood ever so slightly, but to levels that increase the risk for type 2 diabetes and heart disease.

"These disorders have always been with us, but we never saw most of them before because we never had the kinds of foods, the lack of exercise and the aging population that we have today. As these trends continue, it will get even worse," says Dr. Marian Rewers, a preventive medicine expert at the University of Colorado Health Sciences Center, who is tracking the spread of the various forms of diabetes.

Insulin appears to be the key in the development of all forms of diabetes. The foods we eat—an average of two pounds a day of proteins, carbohydrates and fats—are broken down inside our body into glucose and amino acids. Insulin tells cells to snatch glucose from the blood and use it for fuel or store it as fat. Amino acids are used as the building blocks to make cell proteins. As people become fatter, insulin has a harder time doing its job. People with insulin resistance have to produce more insulin than normal to push glucose into muscle and fat cells. When their bodies can't produce enough insulin to get the job done, usually because they have become even fatter, their blood-sugar levels rise and they get diabetes.

People with impaired glucose tolerance are in double jeopardy—they have both too much glucose and too much insulin in their blood. Their body tries to clear excessive glucose by making more insulin and, as a result, their insulin level rises to match their high glucose level. This process sets in motion a cascade of harmful events that lead to high blood pressure, coronary artery disease and type 2 diabetes—in any order and combination. An elevated insulin level seems to be doing things that in the long run are bad for you.

"You're likely to have high blood pressure, high triglycerides, lower HDL cholesterol, changes in blood-clotting factors—a whole series of things linked to excess insulin. It's probably the most common cause of coronary artery disease," says Stanford University's Dr. Gerald Reaven, who coined the term "Syndrome X" to describe the disorders associated with high insulin levels. Three out of four people with diabetes die of heart attacks.

But diabetes can be easily prevented in people who have impaired glucose tolerance. Simply by losing 10 pounds, eating a healthy diet and engaging in moderate physical activity, people with this condition can cut their risk of developing diabetes by about 60 percent. By contrast, overweight people with impaired glucose tolerance who fail to adopt these healthy habits can increase their risk of developing diabetes over a four-year period by 160 percent.

All animals use insulin to exchange food for energy. Humans are the only animals that farm to make food abundant, cook food to make it tasty, elevate meals to an important place in their social life and churn out all kinds of convenience and fast foods that have little relationship to natural products. And humans are the only animals that regularly overeat. You have to force-feed most animals to make them fat.

The trouble in humans starts with what scientists call our thrifty genes. Insulin resistance appears to result from one or more thrifty genes that conferred a survival advantage on our ancestors, who didn't eat very often. Our bodies are designed to be efficient; there's really no way that you can make your body inefficient. But if you stuff more and more food into it, the food eventually has to be converted into fat. If you've got a surfeit of glucose from food, then insulin resistance is simply the phenomenon that results when you can't force anything more into something that's already filled up.

By being insulin resistant, a person quickly banks glucose from a meal into fat deposits, from where it can be tapped for energy in times of want. That was a good strategy for the millions of years of human evolution when food was scarce. But food is always available today. As eating continues nonstop, glucose is stuffed into fat, which accumulates around the waist. This is probably why there's a strong correlation between waistline obesity and the development of diabetes and cardiovascular risk factors.

The new understanding of diabetes tells us that the disease can be prevented and even reversed. But the cure is hard for most people because it requires eating less and becoming more physically active. "In the majority of cases, type 2 diabetes can be corrected if people lose weight and exercise more," says John Lawrence Jr., a Washington University pharmacologist who is studying the harmful effects of too much insulin. "In a sense, there is a cure already out there for most people with diabetes. But most people, like me, can't go on a diet and do it."

Type 2 diabetes can also be controlled with medications that increase the body's production of insulin. However, these drugs lose their effectiveness over a period of about eight years because high glucose levels continue to generate dangerous amounts of free radicals, which, over time, destroy insulin-producing beta cells in the pancreas. People then need to take insulin injections; one out of four adults with diabetes eventually uses insulin.

Antioxidants, however, may be able to halt much of the free radical damage. Dr. Jeffrey Blumberg, an antioxidant expert at Tufts University, calls diabetes a free radical disease. People who have diabetes are chronically deficient in antioxidants. Their bodies quickly use up whatever antioxidants they have to combat the excessive production of free radicals. It is a losing battle: they require more and more antioxidants to prevent escalating free radical damage, just as some people need vitamin C to prevent scurvy or calcium to prevent osteoporosis.

Numerous animal studies show that vitamin E prevents the free radical damage that results from abnormally high blood levels of glucose. And researchers such as Harvard's George King are showing that hefty doses of vitamin E can prevent damage to arteries in the eyes of people with diabetes, thereby greatly reducing their risk of blindness. High doses of the vitamin—1,200 IUs daily—can also reduce the rate of free radical damage to LDL in people with diabetes. The evidence is so compelling that more and more doctors are routinely recommending that their patients with diabetes take vitamin E supplements, in the range of 400 to 800 IUs a day. The vitamin is generally considered safe, but unusually high doses (more than 1,500 IUs) may increase the risk of bleeding in some people.

Using a test that measures levels of antioxidants in the blood, Duke University researchers found that healthy men had twice the antioxidant protection as men with type 2 diabetes. The natural antioxidant defenses of the men with diabetes had fallen precariously low, allowing free radicals to gain the upper hand. In addition, those diabetics with the lowest levels of antioxidants were showing signs of free-radical-induced kidney damage. Based on these studies, Duke's Dr. Emmanuel Opara recommends that people with diabetes increase their intake of such antioxidants as N-acetyl-cysteine and vitamins C and E to block excessive free radical activity.

One promising line of research is the hunt for the genes that make people susceptible to diabetes, genes that behave themselves under normal conditions but misbehave under stresses such as obesity. Scientists also are looking for ways to manipulate genes so people won't become fat even if they overeat, a feat already accomplished in experiments with mice. And, because diabetes in all its forms damages most organ systems of the body, drugs that are effective against this disease also may slow the aging process.

One of the thrifty genes that scientists are tracking down is believed to be a major cause of obesity. Mice with this gene can't control their eating—they eat twice as much as normal mice and get twice as fat. At first, scientists thought the mice got fatter simply because they ate more. But geneticist Edward Leiter of the Jackson Laboratory in Bar Harbor, Maine, found that the thrifty gene bestows an evolutionary advantage on the mice that possess it. By efficiently packing food away as fat, the gene enables the mice to survive in times of scarcity when normal mice would die. When the mice are put on a starvation diet, the normal mice lose weight, become sick and perish. The obese mice, on the other hand, maintain normal body weight and remain healthy on the same restricted diet.

Another gene, called the satiety gene and found in both mice and people, causes obesity in a different way. In its normal form, the gene sends a message to the brain to suppress appetite when sufficient food is consumed. In mice with a defective form of the satiety gene, the brain does not receive the signal and the mice keep eating, becoming up to five times fatter than normal mice. These two genes and others like them are probably what make the Pima Indians and many other people able to survive in a healthy state on a near-starvation diet, but quickly become obese and prone to diabetes when food is plentiful.

The hope for better treatment lies in the development of new drugs that may be able to stop the disease process at the beginning. Two of the most promising drugs—insulin-like growth factor (IGF-1) and troglitazone—appear to be able to prevent insulin resistance, one of the starting points of diabetes. IGF-1 is almost a carbon copy of insulin and it can do many of insulin's jobs. The chemical, however, is better than insulin at converting glucose into muscle instead of fat. The data so far suggest that IGF-1 can reduce blood glucose and lower insulin and it seems to improve blood fats such as cholesterol to levels that reduce the risk of premature cardiovascular disease. When given to people with type 2 diabetes, IGF-1 improves their condition and preliminary findings indicate that it can reverse severe insulin resistance.

Another compound, called insulin-like growth factor-2 (IGF-2), may be able to reduce or prevent damage to peripheral nerves, which affects 10 percent of people with diabetes. Whereas IGF-1 promotes general growth of body tissue, IGF-2 stimulates the repair of damaged nerves. Nerve damage, or diabetic neuropathy—which causes pain and numbness in the hands, feet and legs—can lead to serious complications such as impotence, urinary and bowel dysfunction and gangrene (which results in 50,000 complete or partial amputations annually).

Troglitazone, a promising Japanese anti-diabetes compound, improves the ability of cells to respond to insulin. How it works is not known, but early results show it to be effective in preventing type 2 diabetes. "After we saw that the drug worked so well in diabetics, we thought that maybe it would work in people before they got diabetes, people who are insulin resistant—and it did," says endocrinologist Dr. Jerrold Olefsky of the University of California at San Diego.

Both of these drugs will require further testing to determine if they are safe and effective for treating diabetes and its precursor conditions. Other drugs also are being tested, including antioxidants, which neutralize free radicals and aminoquanadine, which appears to prevent damage caused by high levels of glucose.

Like other free radical diseases, diabetes is being understood at the molecular level. With this growing knowledge comes the power to prevent and reverse this modern epidemic that has made children its newest victims.

# 7

# Preventing Alzheimer's Disease

Every day, Dr. Zaven Khachaturian swallows a golden soft-gel capsule containing 400 IUs of vitamin E; he believes it will reduce his risk of Alzheimer's disease. And he should know—Khachaturian is responsible for much of the research under way to find the cause of and cure for Alzheimer's disease.

When Khachaturian was at the National Institute on Aging, he coaxed bright young scientists into studying Alzheimer's disease, which was considered a dead-end endeavor at the time. But now, that research is beginning to pay off. Khachaturian oversaw the studies showing that people who regularly consume vitamin E have a lower risk of developing Alzheimer's disease. He has also monitored research revealing why the vitamin might work—by neutralizing free radicals before they can sabotage the brain.

Should people start taking vitamin E supplements in their 20s, 30s or 40s to head off a disease that may not strike until they are in their 70s or 80s?

"I'm constantly being asked that question," says Khachaturian, who is now in charge of the Alzheimer's Association's Ronald and Nancy Reagan Research Institute. "On one side, I have to be the rational, heartless bureaucrat who says we need to do more clinical trials to prove once and for all if vitamin E works. But my pragmatic side says that if vitamin E doesn't do any harm, why not take it? People ask me if I take vitamin E and I tell them that I do. They ask if I recommend it to my wife and I tell them that I do.

"We know that vitamin E doesn't cause any problems. We know that there is some indication that it's helpful. So, if you want to take vitamin E as a personal choice, do it in consultation with your physician."

Neurobiologist Mark Mattson believes he knows another sure way to substantially reduce the risk of Alzheimer's disease and, like Khachaturian, he's doing something about it for himself. Evidence from his studies on animals and research from other laboratories indicates that calories do count, especially as an igniting force in neurodegenerative disorders. Essentially, eating too much food stimulates the body to produce excessive amounts of free radicals, which kill brain cells. Low-calorie diets, appreciated for their wondrous anti-aging effects in studies on animals, have now been shown to prevent Alzheimer's disease, Parkinson's and Huntington's disease in mice.

Scientists knew that calorie restriction reduced free radical production, but Mattson's research at the University of Kentucky shows that a low intake of calories protects the brain by turning on a little-understood built-in survival system. Brain cells respond to low calorie consumption by building more antioxidant defenses, bolstering the repair of genes that have been damaged by free radicals and preventing brain cells from dying prematurely.

"When you see that kind of awesome protection, you become a believer," says Mattson. So striking are the safeguards that Mattson has drastically cut back his own calorie consumption, from between 2,500 and 3,000 calories a day to 2,000. He eats more vegetables and less meat and other high-fat foods.

Interestingly, being overweight is not necessarily a risk factor for Alzheimer's disease. Two people can eat the same number of calories but one will put on weight while the other remains thin. This is because their metabolisms differ. Former President Ronald Reagan, who was diagnosed with Alzheimer's disease in his early 80s, was never overweight but he was a voracious eater. A person who eats like that may look normal, but he or she is generating lots of free radicals and increasing his or her risk of Alzheimer's.

After scaring the daylights out of us in 1989 when they told us we were all doomed to get Alzheimer's disease if we lived long enough, scientists such as Mattson and Khachaturian have mounted a spectacular effort to lift that medical curse. They are finding the causes of Alzheimer's and discovering new experimental treatments to delay or prevent it. The study that sounded the Alzheimer's alarm began in 1983 with 3,800 people in East Boston, who continue to be followed today. Scientists have found that, far from being the rare disease it was long thought to be, Alzheimer's is, in fact, quite common, victimizing more than four million Americans. The incidence escalates rapidly with age, affecting one in 10 people over 65 and one in two over 85.

"Ten years ago, the idea of protecting the brain against these degenerative processes was unthinkable," says Dr. Thomas N. Chase, chief of the National Institute on Neurodegenerative Disorders and Stroke's experimental therapeutics branch. "Now the whole field is exploding. The outlook is that we will come up with something to slow down these processes."

**Current attempts to treat Alzheimer's disease are like trying to save the Titanic after it has collided with the iceberg. But now we are developing the knowledge to steer the brain away from the obstacles that can destroy it—free radicals, generally accepted as the root cause of Alzheimer's disease. Although Alzheimer's disease may have a number of different starting points, each ends up increasing free radical damage. The destruction of brain cells by free radicals is a slow process, taking place over a period of 20 to 40 years. Understanding this process opens up the possibility of developing new strategies for preventing the disease, which may be easier than anyone imagined.**

"There's no doubt that excessive amounts of free radicals cause damage to brain cells and that this damage is linked to all types of neurodegenerative diseases," says Khachaturian. "And the list of things that can generate free radicals keeps growing."

Antioxidants such as vitamins C and E are foremost on the list of substances that can help us keep our brains healthy as we age. Treating people with vitamins C and E could be a relatively simple and very safe kind of intervention to delay symptoms of Alzheimer's disease and dementia and sharpen mental acuity into old age. Researchers are hopeful that they will develop treatments to postpone symptoms of Alzheimer's for five or 10 years and eventually prevent the disease altogether.

Giving Alzheimer's patients two widely available compounds—vitamin E and selegiline—demonstrates for the first time that the devastating progression of Alzheimer's disease can be slowed by about 50 percent. Vitamin E and selegiline are both potent antioxidants, adding further evidence to the theory that free radicals cause the death of brain cells. (Selegiline is commonly prescribed under the brand name Eldepryl to treat Parkinson's disease by reducing oxidative stress in the brain.)

People in the two-year study, all of whom had been diagnosed with Alzheimer's disease for an average of five years, were given 1,000 IUs of vitamin E twice a day (more than 100 times the RDA), 5 milligrams of selegiline twice a day, a combination of the two compounds, or a placebo. Vitamin E and selegiline, when taken separately or together, produced significant benefits. The people who took vitamin E or selegiline were better able than those in the placebo group to take care of themselves and to perform daily tasks such as eating, grooming themselves, using the toilet and handling money. They retained more cognitive function, such as remembering lists, and they progressed to severe dementia more slowly. In general, they had a better quality of life than those in the comparison group and they lived longer.

So convincing is the data that the Alzheimer's Disease Cooperative Study researchers, headed by Dr. Leon Thal of the University of California at San Diego, tell doctors they should consider putting patients with moderate Alzheimer's disease on vitamin E or selegiline therapy. The study breaks new ground because for the first time the focus has switched from treating the symptoms of the disease to preventing it. The Alzheimer's Disease Cooperative Study group has launched a massive study to evaluate vitamin E's effectiveness at preventing full-blown Alzheimer's disease in people who have mild memory problems. Since up to 60 percent of these people eventually develop Alzheimer's, the researchers should know fairly conclusively within a few years if vitamin E protects the brain from the destructive processes set in motion by free radicals.

Evidence that vitamin E is a mighty memory saver continues to accumulate. A nationwide study of more than 4,800 elderly Americans found that those who had the highest levels of vitamin E in their blood had the best memories—at any age, from 60 to over 90, and in all racial and ethnic groups.

"Older Americans ought to discuss taking vitamin E with their doctors," says Indiana University School of Medicine biostatistician Siu Hui. The memory tests given the elderly study participants were not based on how much education they had but on their ability to recall newly learned information. Nevertheless, education turned out to be an indicator of how much vitamin E people consumed. People with more than 12 years of education had levels of vitamin E in their blood that were 50 percent higher than those of people who had 10 years or fewer of education and they had superior memories.

Education and vitamin E intake go hand in hand. Vitamin E is one of the few vitamins that cannot be adequately supplied by foods (such as wheat germ oil, peanut oil, corn oil, olive oil and almonds). Educated people have much higher levels of the vitamin because 78 percent of them take vitamin E supplements, either alone or as part of a multivitamin pill. Only 14 percent of the least educated people, those with the lowest vitamin E levels and the poorest memories, take vitamin supplements.

Scientists at the University of Oxford in England found that low levels of two B vitamins—folate (folic acid) and vitamin B-12—are common among people with Alzheimer's disease. Low levels of these two compounds produce high levels of homocysteine in the blood. At high levels, homocysteine is a threat because it becomes a generator of free radicals. (Homocysteine overload has also been added to the list of risk factors for heart disease.) Of 76 Alzheimer's patients in the Oxford study, three out of four had abnormally low levels of folate and vitamin B-12 when compared with healthy people the same age. And their homocysteine levels were dangerously high.

Folate and vitamin B-12 act indirectly as antioxidants by lowering homocysteine levels, thereby curbing the production of free radicals. Routinely testing people for high homocysteine levels and prescribing folate and B-12 to bring homocysteine down to the normal range may serve a dual purpose—protecting against both Alzheimer's and heart disease.

Preventing Alzheimer's disease looks more and more possible as the protective role of antioxidants becomes clearer. A potent mix of antioxidants found in ginkgo biloba extract, an ancient Chinese herbal remedy, produces modest improvements in people with Alzheimer's disease. In a study of Alzheimer's patients who received either the extract or a placebo, the ginkgo mixture was found to be safe and appeared to stabilize or improve the cognitive performance and social functioning of people with dementia. The improvements were significant enough to be recognized by caregivers. Scientists speculate that the synergistic behavior of the main ginkgo antioxidants—flavonoids, terpenoids and organic acids—scavenge the free radicals that assault the brains of Alzheimer's patients. The ginkgo extract, which has long been used in Europe to treat dementia, is made from the leaves, nuts and branches of the ginkgo biloba tree.

Surprisingly, drinking alcohol, as long as it is done in moderation, also protects the brain. Just as antioxidants in wine reduce the risk of heart disease, moderate consumption of alcohol (one drink a day for women and two drinks for men) may lower the risk of Alzheimer's disease by 33 percent. A large Boston University study of older people with dementia also found that drinking slightly more than this amount reduced the

Alzheimer's risk by 52 percent when compared with not drinking at all. According to Lindsay A. Farrer, who conducted the study, the protective effect of alcohol—whether it's in the form of wine, beer or liquor—may come from its ability to quench free radicals, stimulate brain cell repair or prevent mini-strokes. When the researchers balanced out risk factors such as smoking, education and diet, only alcohol stood out as a protective force.

However, Farrar cautions, "It is premature to recommend moderate alcohol consumption as a prophylaxis until the protective mechanism is understood and further studies are performed to more precisely define the minimum level and duration of exposure necessary to realize a benefit."

Chronic inflammation in the brain, which generates free radicals, is another cause of Alzheimer's disease. People who take anti-inflammatory medications for arthritis or other immune disorders have a lower risk of Alzheimer's. Inflammation may trigger Alzheimer's disease when it affects microglia—brain support cells that fight viruses and bacteria, help repair injured cells and eliminate dead tissue. When microglia become chronically inflamed, as they can from a long-lasting infection, they spew out a steady stream of free radicals. Under normal conditions, microglia fire short bursts of free radicals to destroy invading viruses.

However, when the bursts turn into constant torrents, free radicals endanger the nearby neurons that make thought possible. This process seems to occur in people with Down syndrome, who tend to develop Alzheimer's at a young age. Abnormal gene function in the extra copy of chromosome 21 that causes the disorder appears to cause microglia to secrete excessive amounts of free radicals, leading to the death of brain cells.

"Microglia really have killing power," says neuroscientist Carol A. Kincaid-Colton of the Georgetown University School of Medicine, who conducted the research on Down syndrome. "When you look at Alzheimer's brain tissue, you find footprints of free radical damage. As we age, our brains burn up."

A study of mice with Down syndrome found that the mice are ravaged by three times the normal level of free radicals, which helps explain the physical abnormalities and mental retardation that are characteristic of the disease. Preliminary evidence indicates that these abnormalities may be prevented by giving pregnant mice whose fetuses carry the abnormal triple chromosome a drug that boosts a potent natural antioxidant called glutathione. Glutathione can be increased by the drug N-acetyl cysteine, which easily penetrates the brain and other tissues.

"The data are just sitting their screaming at you, 'This is the case, this is the case—it's free radicals and antioxidants!'" says Kincaid-Colton.

Brain cells are built to last more than 100 years. But as free radical damage builds up, the cells die off—starting at age 45 in people with early-onset Alzheimer's. The disease, which can be accurately diagnosed only after death, is marked by the build-up of plaques and tangles in the brain and a dramatic reduction in the number of brain cells. The plaques are made up of cell debris called amyloid beta. Many scientists believe that amyloid beta plaques somehow cause the death of brain cells and many drug companies are trying to develop drugs to prevent the plaques from forming. But the idea that amyloid plaques are the major killers of brain cells leaves many important questions unanswered: extensive plaques can be found in the brains of old people with clear minds who have not experienced brain cell loss, while some people with obvious Alzheimer's symptoms have no plaques in the presence of widespread loss of brain cells.

Scientists at the University of South Florida have discovered how amyloid beta is involved in Alzheimer's disease. Amyloid beta's parent compound is amyloid precursor protein (APP). When it's working properly, APP nurtures brain cells, keeping them healthy and helping to repair them when they are injured. But when APP is mutated, it forms amyloid beta, which turns it into a free radical spitball machine. Exposing living blood vessels from animal brains to small amounts of amyloid beta, the researchers found that the defective protein generates massive amounts of free radicals from the vessel walls and causes the vessels to constrict.

It's a double whammy: free radicals cause more damage to cells and proteins around them and constricted vessels starve brain cells of essential nutrients. Brain cells begin to die. A vicious cycle sets in: more APP is made in an attempt to repair the damage to brain cells, but the excessive generation of free radicals blasts APP apart, forming the injurious amyloid beta protein.

"At first, APP production is a protective mechanism that works in favor of the cell," says Dr. Michael Mullan, head of South Florida's molecular biology lab. "But with age, you have too many free radicals and then the formation of amyloid beta does more damage to brain cells."

The Florida researchers discovered the key to preventing damage from amyloid beta—a naturally occurring antioxidant called superoxide dismutase. Treating blood vessels with superoxide dismutase before exposing them to amyloid beta completely protected the vessels from free radical harm and constriction. "This really opens up the possibility of using antioxidants to delay or prevent Alzheimer's disease," says Mullan.

If amyloid beta could be removed from the brain or prevented from accumulating, then a big source of free radicals could be eliminated and at least some cases of Alzheimer's disease prevented. This is exactly what a group of California scientists accomplished in mice, paving the way for a possible vaccine against Alzheimer's disease in people. The mice are genetically engineered to carry the defective amyloid beta gene in their brain cells. As the mice age they develop a type of dementia that closely resembles Alzheimer's. Performing an experiment that they describe as "we really don't know why we did it," the researchers injected the mice with the amyloid beta protein and a chemical that stimulates the immune system. At first they couldn't believe their eyes—so they threw out the results and started over. But the findings were the same: mice injected with the amyloid beta vaccine when they were young never developed Alzheimer's disease as they aged.

Even more startling, the vaccine stopped the progression of Alzheimer's disease in older mice and caused amyloid plaques in their brains to shrink.

Why? If amyloid beta already exists in the brain, why doesn't the body wipe it out before it can do any harm? No one knows for sure, but it may be that the brain is so protected that the immune system does not normally mount an attack there. By injecting the amyloid beta protein into the blood, the body sees it as an enemy and generates antibodies to destroy it. These same antibodies then travel into the brain to eliminate the protein from there.

Once free radical injury gets out of control and damage occurs faster than brain cells can repair it, another deadly step is activated: chemicals leak from cells, creating a poisonous environment. One of these leaking chemicals is glutamate, a messenger that ordinarily tells brain cells when to turn on to talk to other cells. When it reaches toxic levels, however, glutamate acts as a stun gun, causing cells to spasmodically open doors on their surfaces and allow hyperactive calcium to pour in. Calcium, normally under tight control, triggers a shower of free radical sparks that precipitates a deadly condition called excitotoxicity, driving brain cells to the limits of their endurance. Beaten and battered by free radicals from within and without, the cells succumb. Special genes kick in that force the cells to commit suicide. When they die, depending on their location in the brain, they cause memory to dissolve, muscles to weaken, sanity to flee and life to ebb away.

Because of the important role of free radicals in causing the brain to malfunction, scientists are attempting to devise tests to measure their activity. One test that appears promising uses aspirin, which circulates in the brain and absorbs free radicals. Extracting a tiny amount of cerebral fluid from the spine, where the fluid drains from the brain, scientists can measure the amount of aspirin that has been oxidized by free radicals. Early results show that the spinal fluid of a 70-year-old has 10 times more free radical damage than that of a 30-year-old, says John Carney of the University of Kentucky, who developed the aspirin test with Robert A. Floyd of the Oklahoma Medical Research Foundation. The test could be a way to measure the risk of neurodegenerative damage from free radicals, as well as to determine the effectiveness of antioxidants and other therapies.

Carney believes that he can pep up flagging brains in older people with an antioxidant called PBN. In an experiment on older mice, Carney used PBN to reduce the production of free radicals in their brains to a youthful level. Without a constant bombardment by free radicals, the brain cells were given an opportunity to repair themselves. Learning and memory capabilities in Carney's older animals improved to levels found in young mice. Carney believes that drugs made from PBN will work for people with Alzheimer's disease and he has launched a pharmaceutical company to develop them.

There is even hope for people who have lost brain cells or had them damaged through neurodegenerative processes. Fred Gage of the Salk Institute and Mark Tuszynski of the University of California at San Diego have restored learning and memory in monkeys that had a form of Alzheimer's disease. The astonishing feat was accomplished by genetically engineering skin cells from the monkeys with a gene that makes nerve growth factor (which keeps brain cells alive) and then implanting the cells into the sites in their brains that were being attacked by Alzheimer's. The growth factor spared the lives of endangered cells.

In their search for ways to prevent and reverse brain deterioration, scientists are also tapping into the recently discovered ability of the brain to make new neurons. For 100 years medical textbooks have been saying that the brain didn't make new cells—it only lost them. That the brain has a secret source of renewal provides enormous hope for rebuilding it when necessary. Scientists have already achieved some measure of success in stimulating animal brains to make new neurons to replace missing ones.

We may even be able to increase the production of new brain cells in relatively simple ways such as exercising and learning. The more we engage in physical exercise and mental exercise through learning, the more neurons our brains make to lay down new memory and keep Alzheimer's at bay. The trick to keeping these new brain cells is to lock them in place with experience.

Wouldn't it be nice to learn that a walk around the block could generate thousands, perhaps millions, of new neurons and that you could solidify them by reading a book or working a crossword puzzle? Instead of brain cell transplants, we may find ways to accelerate our own production of brain cells to ward off Alzheimer's and other equally devastating neurodegenerative disorders.

*8*

# Hormones:
# Nature's Rejuvenators

Every day, invisible streams of hormones ebb and flow throughout your body, telling muscles to stay in shape, your brain to be alert, your immune defenses to be on guard and your organs to function flawlessly—in other words, to do their best to keep you healthy.

Because of their ability to carry messages to cells in different parts of the body, hormones have been assigned a number of important jobs, one of the most critical of which is defusing free radicals. Many hormones, it turns out, are potent antioxidants. As they deliver messages to cells, they also act as firemen, putting out free radical sparks along the way or preventing situations from occurring that generate free radicals. Hormones serve double duty—orchestrating cell harmony and minimizing free radical damage to cells and their genetic command posts.

For several decades scientists have painstakingly tracked these elusive chemicals to find out what happens when estrogen, testosterone, growth hormone, melatonin and other hormones decline with age. The evidence is compelling that, as the levels of hormones fall, their power to maintain youthful vigor also subsides. This decline is accompanied by the common signposts of aging—loss of muscle and lean body mass; increase of fat (around the waist for men, the buttocks for women); increased risk of heart disease, cancer, dementia and infections; bone loss; and growing frailty.

Until recently, scientists weren't sure whether hormones decline as a result of aging, or if their decline precedes aging and is, in fact, a major contributor. It appears that the glands that secrete hormones—the pituitary, adrenals, hypothalamus, thymus, ovaries and testicles—gradually suffer the same destruction from free radicals as other body tissues do. As the damage piles up, the ability of the glands to make hormones subsides.

Can aging be retarded by restoring these hormones to the protective levels of young adulthood? Although the question seems obvious, the answer has been hard to come by. Until recently, hormones were difficult to study because they were in short supply and little understood. Drug companies ignored them because they couldn't patent them. With little hope of recouping their investment and making a profit, the pharmaceutical giants resisted spending millions of dollars on research. But many of these companies are now changing their minds as they see the aging of the generation of baby boomers, a population that would welcome rejuvenating compounds if they work. Furthermore, drug companies are quickly developing the skills to invent patentable synthetic chemicals that mimic the activity of natural hormones.

Most hormones are produced in miniscule amounts and their levels in the body fluctuate throughout the day. To get just a couple of drops of a hormone, scientists used to have to process hundreds of thousands of animal glands. This bottleneck was broken only recently when molecular biologists discovered ways to genetically engineer bacteria to make scarce human hormones in bulk. Using this new supply of hormones, scientists are beginning to find some of the answers to the hormone mystery. No one yet knows if hormone supplements will enable us to live significantly longer, but there are tantalizing indications that hormones may be able to increase average life expectancy. Evidence in animals shows that restoring key hormones to more youthful levels can halt and even reverse the effects of aging.

Unlike most hormones, which decline with age, some hormones such as insulin (which regulates cell metabolism) and leptin (which regulates appetite) tend to increase with age. As the cells that are the normal targets of these hormones grow older, they no longer respond to the hormones. A failing response to insulin causes more of the hormone to be produced, leading to a buildup of glucose in the blood and diabetes. A failing response to leptin leads to weight gain.

Leptin is secreted by fat cells and travels to receptors in the brain when a fatty meal has been eaten to signal the brain to turn down appetite and aid metabolism. But as the aging brain cells fail to respond, the body increases leptin production in a futile attempt to tell the brain that the body has enough fat. With the lines of communication broken, appetite goes unchecked and fat cells are forced to gobble up more fat than they should. Preliminary evidence suggests that giving obese people extra amounts of leptin may break this logjam by reopening the communication lines to the brain, helping them to control their weight.

Many people unwittingly tamper with their hormones by cheating on their sleep. Scientists are finding that skimping on slumber plays havoc with important hormones, potentially endangering brain cells, depleting the immune system and promoting the growth of fat instead of muscle. Chronic sleep deprivation may be as dangerous to health as eating a bad diet or being sedentary, and it can accelerate the aging process. Yet most Americans, bombarded by increasing demands on their time from work, travel, leisure activities, family responsibilities and social obligations, steal time from sleep.

To find out what lack of slumber does to the body's hormones, University of Chicago sleep researcher Eve Van Cauter takes around-the-clock blood samples from volunteers, both when they are awake and when they're asleep. (A plastic tube attached to a needle in a vein allows the researchers to take blood samples from another room without disturbing a subject's sleep.) Van Cauter's findings raise red flags. Lack of sleep causes blood levels of the stress hormone cortisol to go up, while levels of two other important hormones—muscle-building human growth hormone and immune-boosting prolactin—go down. These reactions are just the opposite of what they should be. Staying awake longer than normal may be at the cost of stress-related memory impairment, increased risk of infection and more flab.

Cortisol poses the biggest danger. Normally, the hormone declines at night to prepare the body for sleep and increases in the morning to make a person alert for the day's activities. Limiting sleep to four hours instead of eight for just one night can cause cortisol levels to remain high the next day and through the next night. At stressful times, the adrenal glands release cortisol to prepare the body to temporarily cope with the stress; production of the hormone subsides once the stressful event is over. The hormone is so powerful that the body turns it off when it is not needed. Studies on older people show that long-term exposure to abnormally high levels of cortisol can damage brain cells directly, shrinking the hippocampus, a critical region of the brain that regulates learning and memory. The increase in evening cortisol levels can impair memory if it occurs regularly as a result of chronic sleep deprivation.

"People think they can lose sleep and they'll be tired, but otherwise they'll be fine," says Van Cauter. "This is the first study to show that this isn't true. In addition to the effects on mood and alertness, chronic voluntary sleep curtailment may have long-term adverse health effects and it is likely to accelerate aging."

When Van Cauter deprived a group of young men of sleep for six nights, she found an ominous change in their hormone patterns. In many ways, their hormone profile was in tatters, looking like that of men in their 60s. Allowing the volunteers to sleep 12-hour periods restored their hormones to youthful levels. This kind of recuperative power diminishes as people get older and their periods of deep sleep—the time when they make key brain hormones—naturally shorten.

As more hormones are put into pill form, expectations rise that they may provide a simple way to prolong youth. But for all of their promise, hormone supplements, except for estrogen, have yet to be proven safe and effective over the long term. Because they seem to be nature's own antidote to aging, it is easy for hucksters to oversell them with unrealistic promises. Melatonin, for example, may or may not slow aging. It is an active antioxidant and it can reset the body's sleep cycle, which is especially helpful for jet lag. But some parents are wading into dangerous waters by giving their infants melatonin to help them sleep at night. The danger is that melatonin supplements could prevent an infant's own hormone system from developing properly. In this case and possibly others, the unwise use of hormones could cause more harm than good.

"Some of these hormones are going to be useful against some aspects of aging," predicts Richard L. Sprott, chief of the National Institute on Aging's Biology of Aging program. "We will find therapies that reduce the incidence or severity of the long-term debilitating diseases that characterize the latter part of the life span, but I don't think we've got the fountain of youth. We have a real concern that people not get accustomed to the notion that they're going to get better health and a longer life by taking a pill rather than by making the kind of lifestyle changes, such as exercise and a good diet, that we know actually do make a difference. Wrinkles, for example, are totally preventable if you keep your skin out of the sun and don't smoke."

Sometimes it's hard to restrain enthusiasm when preliminary findings suggest wonderful improvements. This is the case with DHEA. Known scientifically as dehydroepiandrosterone, DHEA is produced in the adrenal glands and starts to decline after about age 20. Once ignored as an inconsequential hormone, DHEA has become a potential superstar. DHEA was thought at first to have only one role—to make the sex hormones, estrogen and testosterone. Scientists have since discovered a second, equally important role: on its own, DHEA seems to protect against many of the diseases that go hand-in-hand with aging in some people.

When Samuel S. C. Yen at the University of California at San Diego gave eight men and eight women over age 50 DHEA supplements to bring the hormone up to peak levels, he was startled by the results. "Their ability to cope with day-to-day stress increased. They had an increased quality of sleep, decreased joint pain and increased joint mobility. They feel happy," he says. Yen and other experts stress that large, long-term studies are needed to verify the preliminary findings.

Among other things, DHEA seems to placate unruly immune systems that turn against the body, a major cause of autoimmune diseases such as rheumatoid arthritis and lupus. A three-month study of 28 women has shown that taking 200 milligrams of DHEA daily helps to control the symptoms of lupus. Autoimmune diseases are doubly troublesome: not only does the inflammatory response they cause chew up joints and other tissues, it also generates excessive amounts of free radicals, which add to the destruction. DHEA comes to the rescue of the body by curbing free radical production and down-regulating the inflammatory response. Instead of blotting up free radicals, as most antioxidants do, DHEA prevents these destructive particles from ever forming.

Newer findings suggest that the brain makes its own supply of DHEA, which it uses to grow new connections between brain cells. When scientists at the University of California at San Francisco gave DHEA to older people who had low levels of the hormone, their memories improved and so did their psychological well-being and mood.

The major drawback of DHEA supplements is that the hormone eventually gets converted into estrogen and testosterone. Too much of either of these sex hormones can cause trouble: estrogen causes breast enlargement in men and testosterone causes excessive growth of facial hair in women. To overcome these problems, scientists are developing look-alike drugs that have the beneficial effects of DHEA without its side effects. One of these compounds is already undergoing early clinical trials for cancer, diabetes and arthritis.

Careful testing of hormones is necessary to avoid the pitfalls that occurred when estrogen was first approved for use. Estrogen replacement therapy was in urgent demand in the 1960s because elderly women were developing osteoporosis at a fast rate and breaking their bones in falls. Hip fractures were the most common reason women were admitted to nursing homes and the cause of many deaths. Giving women estrogen supplements stemmed the epidemic of fractures. But after more than 10,000 women had taken the compound, scientists noticed that the women had an increased risk of uterine cancer. Progesterone, another sex hormone, was added to estrogen therapy to counteract the effects of estrogen on the uterus and reduce the small risk of uterine cancer.

Later there seemed to be a link between estrogen supplements and a slightly increased risk of breast cancer, but this link remains marginal. In fact, women who are at risk of developing breast cancer and take the supplement live longer than women with similar breast-cancer risk who don't take estrogen. The essential point is that even naturally-occurring body chemicals may cause problems when used in unusual ways. This is why long-term testing of hormones is crucial before they are put into widespread use. Now that hundreds of thousands of women have used estrogen supplements for long periods, the evidence is overwhelmingly in favor of the hormone as a lifesaver.

Estrogen does many things, from blocking free radicals to lowering LDL (the cholesterol that increases the risk of heart disease) and elevating HDL (the cholesterol that protects against heart disease). Women ages 70 to 74 are four times more likely to die of heart disease than breast cancer. The Nurses Health Study has shown that the risk of dying from a heart attack is 53 percent lower and dying from all causes is 37 percent lower in women taking estrogen supplements than in women who are not taking the hormone.

Most recently, estrogen is being given together with parathyroid hormone to build strong new bone in the spine and hip and reverse the progression of osteoporosis. Women who take this combination therapy have a dramatically lower risk of fractures. Estrogen also works in the brain, nurturing neurons and protecting them against free radical damage. Women who take estrogen supplements are half as likely to develop Alzheimer's disease as women who don't take estrogen. In the future, doctors may even recommend that men take estrogen, or some version of it, to protect their brains, since the male brain naturally makes small amounts of the hormone.

To take advantage of estrogen's enormous benefits, drug makers are devising "designer" estrogens, compounds called SERMs (selective estrogen-receptor modulators), which do all of the good deeds of estrogen without affecting the breast or uterus. One of these SERMs, raloxifene, appears to have all of estrogen's good characteristics and none of its bad ones. The compound slows bone loss and has been approved for preventing osteoporosis. Scientists tracking raloxifene's ability to improve bones were little prepared for the discovery of what is perhaps raloxifene's biggest benefit: it reduces the risk of breast cancer by up to 70 percent. Raloxifene also increases blood levels of HDL, just as estrogen does, and it may protect women against heart disease. An additional bonus—raloxifene does not increase the risk of uterine cancer.

The latest rush to tap into the potential rejuvenating powers of hormones started in the early 90s when the late Dr. Daniel Rudman of the Medical College of Wisconsin in Milwaukee reported that growth hormone injections given to healthy men ages 61 to 85 built their muscles and melted fat away. It was the first bona fide scientific experiment to reverse aging with hormones. Other researchers have found similar results, but they have also discovered that, by itself, growth hormone has some drawbacks. While growth hormone increases lean body mass and decreases fat deposits, it generally does not increase muscle strength. And it can have side effects such as carpal tunnel syndrome and swelling. The only group to increase strength and psychological well-being from growth hormone supplements are young men who do not produce enough of their own growth hormone but have normal levels of other hormones.

The problem is that in all of the experiments done so far, subjects have been given a big dose of the hormone once a day. The pituitary normally secretes much smaller amounts of growth hormone four or five times a day. To copy this natural pattern, new drugs are being developed that stimulate the pituitary to secrete small bursts of growth hormone throughout the day. These drugs are likely to be more effective than the large hormone injections.

Insulin-like growth factor (IGF-1) is another hormone that may be able to make an old body vigorous again. If successful experiments in rats can be transferred to humans, an 80-year-old could regain the muscle mass and strength of a 30-year-old. University of Pennsylvania researchers, headed by physiologist H. Lee Sweeney, were able to produce this remarkable feat in rodents using gene therapy. Encapsulating the IGF-1 gene into a harmless cold virus and injecting it into the muscles of young and old rats, they achieved an amazing increase in strength. The young rats increased their strength by 15 percent but old rats, which, like humans, lose one-third of their muscle as they age, gained back nearly 30 percent of their strength and were as strong as the young rats. The IGF-1 gene appears to work by stimulating the production of new muscle cells to replace dying ones, a potential boon for people with muscle-wasting diseases such as muscular dystrophy and amyotrophic lateral sclerosis (ALS).

Like other hormone-replacement experiments, this one shows that the body retains great reserves as it ages, but that even minor free radical damage can slow the body's production of hormones. With a little extra effort, such as equipping muscle cells with fresh insulin-like growth factor genes, many of these crucial hormones can be switched on again.

But the use of drugs to increase strength and decrease fat may be unnecessary for many older people. Several studies have shown that the level of growth hormone can become depleted simply through lack of use—and can be increased with exercise. Frail elderly people who perform daily resistance exercises, such as lifting their legs and arms with small weights, increase their levels of growth hormone and their muscle strength. Even those who have been wheelchair-bound can get up and move about on their own after doing strengthening exercises.

For now, testosterone appears to be the hormone most likely to follow estrogen to FDA approval. The evidence is becoming more persuasive that testosterone may be able to build stronger muscles in people with muscle-wasting and muscle-weakness disorders and even reverse the normal muscle weakening that comes with aging. Although testosterone is thought to be solely a male sex hormone, women also make it, but in smaller amounts. Like estrogen, testosterone is a jack-of-all-trades hormone. In addition to imprinting male characteristics, testosterone appears to play a role in maintaining memory and in regulating other hormones. As testosterone declines, for instance, levels of leptin (the fat-regulating hormone) climb.

The combination of declining testosterone and increasing leptin appears to account for the loss of muscle and increase in fat that plague older men. Restoring testosterone levels causes leptin to decrease, suggesting that fat metabolism is under better control. Adequate levels of testosterone also appear to be necessary for growth hormone to work properly; growth hormone makes muscles grow, but testosterone is necessary to make them stronger. This explains why younger men whose bodies don't make enough growth hormone can build stronger muscles with growth hormone supplements—they are making adequate amounts of testosterone.

Testosterone levels start declining at about age 40 and, by age 80, are only one-third to one-half their peak levels. There is some concern that taking testosterone supplements may carry some potential dangers, such as an increased risk of heart disease or prostate cancer. But a yearlong study by Saint Louis University gerontologist Dr. John E. Morley found no evidence of these risks in men who take testosterone supplements. Blood levels of PSA, a protein that is used to measure prostate cancer risk, did not increase during the trial and the men experienced an increase in strength.

"The men were a lot happier," observes Morley. "If you're 75 years old and falling down, an increase in muscle strength of even three or four percent is a big help."

Older men may be candidates for testosterone replacement therapy if they have experienced decreases in sex drive, energy, strength, enjoyment of life, work performance, height, or if they fall asleep after dinner or are sadder or grumpier than usual. Says Morley, "The significant result of this research is that we will now be able to treat men effectively for male menopause—to help prevent a decline in health due to aging."

So, the answer to the question of whether hormones can retard aging seems to be a qualified "yes." More research is needed for some hormones, but we already have learned how we can manipulate hormones to restore some measure of youth by getting enough sleep, doing strength-building exercises, reducing stress and taking estrogen replacement therapy when appropriate.

## 9

# *Living Longer by Eating Less*

Following in the footsteps of a long line of scientists who have experimented on themselves, Roy Walford has happily adopted the eating pattern of his laboratory mice at the University of California, Los Angeles. For Walford, it's a chance to taste immortality. He saw it happen to his mice: eating a calorie-restricted diet they lived the equivalent of 150 human years. By consuming about 1,800 calories a day since 1987, instead of the 2,000 to 2,800 normally recommended for a male his age, Walford believes he can live at least to the age of 120.

He says he could have increased his potential life span to 140 if he had started eating less food a decade or two earlier. But it wasn't until the late 80s that he and Richard Weindruch of the University of Wisconsin discovered that calorie restriction can prolong life no matter when you start. They also found that the fewer calories you eat, the greater the health benefits. In mice, 10 percent fewer calories increases life by 10 percent, while 40 percent fewer calories means a 40 percent longer life.

Walford, who turned 76 in 2000, firmly believes that humans can double their average life expectancy—now about 76 years—simply by cutting back on food. That means eating a well-balanced diet with about 30 percent fewer calories than you consumed at your best weight, usually around young adulthood. And all calories count, whether they come from fat, a primary source, or carbohydrates and protein; all calories are converted into fat by the body and stored for future energy needs.

Walford likes to point out that calorie restriction is a far better deal than the bargain Faust struck with the devil, trading a mere 24 additional years of youth for an eternity in hell. But is he right? And if long life can be achieved just by eating less, is that something that most people could, or would, do, given the fact that one in three American adults is obese and the majority are overweight to some degree?

Most scientists who study the biology of aging are not willing to go out on the same longevity limb as Walford, at least not yet. They agree, however, that Walford may be on the right track and the federal government is willing to gamble millions of dollars to find out if dietary restriction is really the simplest, fastest and most effective path to living considerably longer in good health. Calorie restriction is seen as a vital key to understanding the aging process because it is the only sure-fire way to dramatically prolong life and youth in all of the small animals it has so far been tried on. Scientists will not know if this is a universal phenomenon until they test it on monkeys and humans, which they are doing. So far the results suggest that calorie restriction may work for us too.

Scientists are fascinated by calorie restriction because it appears to awaken an ancient evolutionary survival mechanism. When food is scarce, which it has been for most of the millions of years of human development, life and reproduction are threatened. To ensure survival under conditions of scarcity, nature built in systems that allow organisms to live a lot longer by delaying growth, maturation and reproduction. An extreme and dangerous example of this phenomenon is anorexia; in women with this disorder, who are on starvation diets, their reproductive system shuts down and they stop menstruating.

But short of starvation, calorie restriction does wondrous things. Metabolism undergoes dramatic changes, turning into a highly protective shield against the onslaught of aging. Hibernation is a common example of how metabolism can keep organisms alive for months and even years when no food is available. Most insects that survive the winter do so by hibernating.

**Calorie restriction upgrades most systems of the body; it jacks up hormone levels, strengthens immune defenses and efficiently replaces**

aged cells with young ones. But the most important contribution of calorie restriction to longevity may be its ability to reduce free radical damage and boost cell repair. When fewer calories are taken in, the body produces fewer free radicals and the free radicals that it makes are mopped up by increased antioxidant defenses. At the same time, free radical damage to DNA and other cell components is repaired more rapidly.

With all this good news about the potential life-prolonging benefits of eating less, it would seem to be an easy strategy to follow. But it's not. People like to eat and they are eating more and more processed and fast foods that tend to have lots of fat and calories. The short-term pleasure of eating a wide variety of foods, never before available in such abundance, is a greater temptation than the long-term and as yet unproven goal of living longer while enduring some degree of hunger.

"Food tastes so darn good," complains Roger McCarter, an expert on calorie restriction and professor of physiology at the University of Texas Health Science Center in San Antonio. "The longevity benefits of calorie restriction are telling us that we eat too much and we exercise too little. It's very simple. We eat a diet that the National Institutes of Health would not allow us to feed to our rats. On average, the fat content of the typical North American diet is 35 percent. It's ridiculous and yet we feed it to our kids. There's a stupidity here that's coming back to bite us."

Even most of the scientists who study calorie restriction find the diet hard to swallow. "My colleagues and I around here have been studying this stuff for about 20 years and there's not a single one of us who's restricting calories," admits McCarter. "Yet the data are compelling. There's no question it works; it's just hard to do."

Scientists are searching for populations of people who, for one reason or another, are eating less. They want to see if food deprivation is prolonging life in humans and improving their health by reducing their risk of cancer, heart disease and other chronic disorders. So far they have found tantalizing hints that this is happening. People who live on the island of Okinawa, for example, whose average age hovers around the mid-80s, live far longer than most people, including other Japanese. Their food intake is 17 percent lower in adults and 36 percent lower in children than the average Japanese. Okinawans have a death rate from cancer, heart disease and stroke that is 31 to 41 percent lower than the Japan national average, which itself is lower than the rate in the U.S.

The Harvard Alumni Health Study and the Nurses Health Study found that deaths from all causes are considerably reduced in people whose weight is 15 to 20 percent below the national average. In another study, 60 elderly people who were put on a food-restricted diet had fewer deaths and hospitalizations over time than a similar group of elderly people who continued to eat as they always had. And a study of nearly 4,000 British children suggests that eating less in adolescence may reduce the risk of cancer later in life. The study, which began in 1937 when the youths were 16 years old, found that, more than 60 years later, those who ate less as teenagers were less likely to die of cancer than were adults who had overeaten in their youth. In all of these studies, cigarette smoking and other risk factors were balanced out.

To find out what calorie restriction does to the body biologically, scientists are studying its effects in monkeys. Monkeys are genetically very close to humans, so if diet restriction works to prolong their lives it will probably work in people too. The National Institute on Aging is employing this strategy on about 200 monkeys at the NIH animal center in Poolesville, Virginia. The primates are divided into two groups; one group is allowed to eat as much as it wants and the second group is given 30 percent less food than what the monkeys would eat if they had free access to food. In both groups, the food is nutritiously balanced. Although it is too early to tell if the food-restricted monkeys are living longer, there is ample evidence that their bodies are doing all the things that long-lived mice do: their metabolism adjusts to a survival mode, utilizing energy more efficiently, reducing free radical damage, tightening stress defenses, repairing cell damage more swiftly and slowing growth and reproduction in favor of survival.

The bodies of the calorie-restricted monkeys seem to be declaring war against heart disease. Their triglycerides (blood fats linked to an increased risk of atherosclerosis) and blood pressure are down, while levels of HDL (the good cholesterol) are up. Another marker of aging, DHEA—a hormone that gives rise to estrogen, testosterone and other compounds—declines at a slower rate in the food-restricted monkeys. Because of the evidence that DHEA may also protect against cancer, immune disorders and heart disease, high levels of the hormone in the food-restricted monkeys may help protect them from these illnesses. Initially, dietary restriction seems to slow metabolism, but after awhile, it adjusts. Within a couple of months of putting monkeys on calorie restriction, they experience about a one-degree drop in body temperature. This indicates a metabolic change whereby they're shifting from growth and reproduction to a life-maintenance strategy.

"I think calorie restriction is working in monkeys and I think that bodes well for having beneficial effects in people," says George Roth, chief of the National Institute on Aging's molecular physiology and genetics section. "The real question in my mind is whether or not people would be willing to stay on a restricted diet. It probably would be better if we could find the mechanism by which dietary restriction works and then develop drugs or something so that we can trick cells into thinking they're restricted without a person having to go on a 30 percent reduced diet."

When UCLA's Walford signed up to be the physician on an eight-person crew that spent two years sealed in Biosphere 2, a space-colony prototype in the Arizona desert, he never dreamed he would have a chance to test calorie restriction in humans. But that's what happened. The crew consisted of four men and four women whose average age was 35, excluding Walford, who was in his 60s. Their goal was to be totally independent of the outside world, as if they were in a space station on Mars or the moon, growing their own food from recycled water and wastes.

"We couldn't raise enough food, as it turned out," Walford grins. "But what we did grow was high quality. We ended up on a calorie-restricted but nutrient-dense diet, exactly the type we use in animals. So I turned it into an experiment. I did a lot of studies on the changes in our blood chemistry, hormones and things like that. On the whole, we behaved exactly the way animals do on that kind of diet."

The diet was primarily vegetarian. The biospherians ate lots of vegetables, grains and legumes, a modest amount of fruit, half a glass of goat milk a day, fish occasionally and meat once a week. Were they content with their frugal diet? The crew members were often hungry, but as long as they were convinced the diet was safe, they were willing to stick with it for the sake of science.

In the long run, they may be glad they did. Their temperature dropped slightly and they lost weight. But what was going on inside their bodies was even more significant: free radical production dropped, antioxidant defenses increased, DNA repair picked up, their immune defenses got stronger, levels of insulin and blood sugar (risk factors for diabetes and other age-related disorders) declined and hormone changes followed the same life-enhancing pattern that occurs in mice and monkeys that are put on restricted diets. Total cholesterol levels dropped from an average pre-entry level of 190 to 130.

"It would be surprising if we had all the same physiologic changes from calorie restriction as animals but didn't get the life span increase," says Walford. He continues to follow the Biosphere crew, taking regular blood samples and monitoring their health. Some have stayed on a restricted diet and they continue to reap its rewards. But among those who resumed their old ways of eating, levels of cholesterol, blood sugar and other bio-chemical markers have crept up and they have lost the physiological improvements they had gained while living in the Biosphere.

One of the benefits of calorie restriction that may make it more palatable to people is that it makes rodents a lot friskier than usual. If they were in the rodent Olympics, they would win all the gold medals. This phenomenon is counterintuitive: animals that eat less should have less energy and just want to lie around. But the opposite is true. Animals that are allowed to eat all they want slow down with age, as people do, and become less active. Animals fed 40 percent less food, on the other hand, engage in a high level of physical activity throughout their lives.

McCarter, of the University of Texas Health Science Center in San Antonio, puts exercise wheels in cages so that the rats can run any time they want. The animals that are fed 40 percent less food run an average of five kilometers a night for just about their whole lives. Rats that eat freely run only about one kilometer a night at their peak, slow down to 500 meters as they grow older and finally stop running altogether.

"The most amazing thing was that at a time when every single freely-eating rat was dead, more than 80 percent of the food-restricted rats were still alive and running five kilometers every night," he says. "The effects were astonishing."

In his studies of how calorie restriction turns rodents into superathletes, McCarter sees biological changes such as reduced free radical production, increased antioxidant levels, and improved cell-repair mechanisms. In addition, the animals' insulin and blood sugar levels decrease, enabling them to use energy more efficiently. All of these very primitive survival mechanisms kick in with dietary restriction.

This is music to Walford's ears. So when people ask, "How can I slow aging?" he now says, "To live longer, you need to eat less and eat more wholesomely. That's it, basically. If you reduce food consumption even a little bit, you increase life a little bit. If you do it more rigorously, you increase it longer. There isn't any threshold and you don't have to starve."

## 10

# *Anti-aging Genes*

It is generally accepted that whites live longer than blacks; that Alzheimer's disease is an equal-opportunity brain destroyer; and that aging is a rapidly progressive downhill ride into frailty and poor health. But as more people are living longer, these notions of aging are being turned upside down. When people reach very old age, they cross a previously unknown threshold, entering a time warp in which aging slows dramatically and the diseases of aging keep their distance.

It's a special time of life that reverses general trends. Blacks who reach the age of 75 tend to live longer than whites; men who live to 85 are in better mental health than women their age; and people who live into their 90s seem to put aging on pause. Centenarians, for example, are generally healthier than people in their 80s: they have escaped the diseases of aging—such as heart disease, diabetes and Alzheimer's disease—that claim their contemporaries at far younger ages. When the end comes, centenarians tend to die quickly after a brief illness.

"Centenarians have a history of aging very slowly and not getting the diseases associated with aging," says Dr. Thomas T. Perls, a gerontologist at Harvard Medical School, who is studying how people get to be 100 years old and older. "Cancer is extremely rare in centenarians. If they develop Alzheimer's disease, it's very late in life, in their mid-90s, which is much later than most people develop it."

When Jeanne Louise Calment died in 1997 at the age of 122, she not only set the world record for the longest-lived human being, she did it in style. Born in 1875 in Arles, France, Calment was 14 when the Eiffel

Tower was completed in Paris. As a young girl she met Vincent Van Gogh when the artist came to purchase art supplies at her uncle's shop. What accounted for Calment's long life? Qualities in her favor were her positive mental attitude, wit and sense of humor. She was also physically active, riding her bicycle until she was 100. She insisted that the special formula for her longevity was olive oil, port wine and a smile. "I've only ever had one wrinkle and I'm sitting on it," she quipped. "I will die laughing."

Perhaps most important were Calment's genes. She was probably blessed with one or more anti-aging genes. Her brother, who died at the age of 97, was equally lucky. Anti-aging genes, which are randomly distributed in the population, protect the fortunate who have them from age-related diseases of the heart, brain and muscles. They confer this protection by reducing damage from free radicals, hastening repair of genes and cells, cleaning up cholesterol in the blood and performing other tasks that keep the body in good health longer. What else could explain Calment's defiance of the odds—eating a rich French diet, consuming two pounds of chocolate weekly, smoking cigarettes until five years before she died and drinking wine regularly?

Scientists suspect that there are many different kinds of anti-aging genes. After directing the construction of a human being, genes turn their energies to maintaining that person's existence. Among the genes that are being found and catalogued in the Human Genome Project, scientists are intensely searching for those they believe account for why the oldest old live so long. These genes could provide the secret to a longer and healthier life for everyone.

**In the average person, genes may be responsible for about one-third of the effects of aging. The other two-thirds is determined by how we live—the food we eat, our level of physical activity and our environment, all of which can affect the critical balance between free radicals and antioxidants. The larger role that lifestyle and environment play is demonstrated by the fact that life expectancy has tripled in the last**

2,000 years. **Our genes didn't change in that blink of time on the evolutionary scale—but the way we live has changed considerably.**

There are an estimated 7,000 to 8,000 genes that not only determine how fast a person ages, but also how susceptible he or she is to the diseases associated with aging. Centenarians are a gold mine for ferreting out anti-aging genes. Of particular interest is a handful of genes that regulate mitochondria, the energy-producing factories in our cells. Mitochondrial genes are typical of nature's double-edged-sword approach to life. On the one hand, mitochondria are absolutely essential because they drive metabolism, converting the food we eat into the energy we need to live. On the other hand, mitochondria produce free radicals as an unavoidable byproduct of energy production.

"A lot of people think that the free radicals you need to worry about are the ones that come from the environment [such as cigarette smoke and radiation from the sun]," Perls says. "The most important free radicals are the ones that you generate in your own body as a result of metabolism and energy production. Some of us are probably a lot more efficient at producing energy with far fewer free radicals."

Centenarians may be doing this. Free radicals are an important part of the aging story, not only in people who produce fewer of them, but also in people who are able to scavenge them better, getting rid of them before they cause harm. Very old people appear to have some genes that operate well above average, providing added defenses against the aging process and the diseases that often tag along. By discovering anti-aging genes, scientists hope to develop new gene therapies, drugs, special vitamin formulas or even combinations of foods that could enhance the activity of these genes and increase life expectancy for everyone.

"Eventually, we will find genetic markers that can be used to identify people who are at high risk of developing Alzheimer's disease," says Perls. "Then, when they're in their 20s we can give them a pill they take for the rest of their lives, which will prevent them from ever developing Alzheimer's. There is evidence that antioxidant therapy helps Alzheimer's patients. Some people are already saying that maybe the children of Alzheimer's patients should start taking vitamin E and other antioxidants in hopes of avoiding the disease."

Perls compares the human body to a car that you can expect to drive for 100,000 miles under normal circumstances. You can add another 100,000 miles with good maintenance; for humans, good maintenance would mean such steps as taking vitamin E and other antioxidants, which may add more healthy years to life. Rough driving and lack of maintenance can subtract 20,000 to 50,000 miles from the life of a car, just as smoking, lack of exercise, a bad diet and other risky habits can drastically shorten life expectancy. If you want your car to go 300,000 miles, you need to have superstrong alloys and long-lasting lubricants; this is what the centenarians seem to have with their longevity genes and healthful lifestyles.

"To get to 100 and beyond, longevity genes are absolutely crucial," says Perls. "When you're talking about average life expectancy, everybody gets to the age of 75. Whether you live a little bit longer or shorter depends on lifestyle risks such as how much fat you eat and health risks such as diabetes. Getting to 100 years is a very different ball of wax."

Genetic engineering may change all of that with the growing ability to transform ordinary genes into anti-aging genes, making it easy and routine to reach 100 and older. Thomas Johnson of the Institute for Behavioral Genetics at the University of Colorado was the first to alter a single gene in the tiny backyard roundworm, C. elegans, to more than double the worm's life span. The worm gene, appropriately named Age-1, appears to grant longevity by subduing free radical damage. If similar genes exist in humans, doubling the human life span sometime in the future may be a reasonable expectation.

The most promising anti-aging approach involves antioxidant genes, which can slow aging and lengthen life span. Using genetic-engineering techniques, scientists have already boosted the life span of fruit flies and C. elegans worms by giving them extra antioxidant genes or turning their own antioxidant genes on high. When Tony Parkes of the University of Guelph, Ontario, Canada, inserted the human gene for the potent antioxidant superoxide dismutase (SOD) into the nerve cells of fruit flies, he watched in wonder as they defied the odds.

Nerve cells, which control the body's muscles and movements, are especially susceptible to free radical damage. Fruit flies armed with the human SOD gene fought off free radicals so effectively that the flies lived an astonishing 40 percent longer than normal. The discovery that a single antioxidant gene could do this was eye opening and may very well point to ways to lengthening the human life span.

While Calment, the celebrated French centenarian, is only presumed to have had an anti-aging gene or two, Helen Boley of Kansas City, Missouri, has a longevity gene that's been identified. Boley came to the attention of researchers by having the highest recorded level of HDL, the beneficial cholesterol. HDL protects against heart disease by removing artery-clogging cholesterol from the blood and from artery walls and carrying it to the liver, which deactivates it and eliminates it from the body.

The so-called bad cholesterol, LDL, transfers cholesterol to cells. In excessive amounts, LDL becomes a target of free radicals; wounded LDL molecules can infiltrate the lining of arteries, causing the build-up of fatty plaques that are the hallmark of heart disease and the forerunner of stroke. HDL protects vulnerable LDL molecules from free radicals. An HDL level above 40 is considered to be protective because it is at that level that cholesterol can be removed faster than it can be deposited as artery plaques.

When Boley's HDL level was measured at age 68, it was an astounding 230. Like Calment, Boley can eat a rich diet—all the meat, eggs, cheese and bacon she wants—and her arteries will remain clean. Whatever it is that endows Boley with the world-record HDL level, she seems to have inherited it. Many of her relatives lived into their 90s and it appears that they never developed heart disease. Taking regular samples of Boley's blood, scientists at the Heart, Lung and Blood Institute discovered Boley's

"Methuselah factor"—a gene called A-1, which directs the manufacture of HDL. Boley has a slight mutation in the gene, which sets its activity on high, causing it to produce HDL at an enormous rate.

"This pointed to a high HDL level clearly being a way in which you could protect against early heart disease," says Dr. Brian Brewer, chief of the institute's molecular disease branch. Rabbits genetically engineered with the same type of A-1 mutation as Boley's were protected against heart disease no matter how much fat they ate. They were hopping around long after similar rabbits without the A-1 mutation were dead from cholesterol-choked arteries.

In their pursuit of the A-1 gene, researchers have stumbled across another gene that also has the power to regulate HDL. Called LCAT, this human gene may have more immediate application in the treatment of heart disease. While A-1 regulates the production of HDL, LCAT determines how efficiently HDL can pick up and discard cholesterol. Studies on rabbits have found that LCAT's ability to scavenge cholesterol provides as much protection against heart disease as the A-1 mutation does. Drugs are now being developed to turn on the LCAT gene, providing a potential new treatment for heart disease.

The search for anti-aging genes could also change the course of Alzheimer's disease. Why is it that some people, like former President Ronald Reagan, grow older with brains increasingly clouded by Alzheimer's disease, while others enter their nineties clear-headed? One reason seems to be the luck of the genetic draw. Many cases of Alzheimer's disease appear to be linked to a family of genes known as apoE. All humans have genes that make proteins for hair, fingernails, blood, and all the other parts of the body. But, while the genes are similar, they come in slightly different forms.

This is the case with the apoE family of genes, which has three varieties—apoE-2, apoE-3 and apoE-4. ApoE is important because it builds proteins that help lipoproteins (such as LDL and HDL) find their targets as they carry cholesterol to and from cells. Nowhere in the body is this more important than in the brain, where cholesterol is in constant use to repair neurons and build new connections between them as learning takes place and memory is laid down. Everyone inherits two apoE genes, one from each parent, so the genes can come in six different combinations.

About 65 percent of the population possess two apoE-3 genes, which give them an average risk of developing Alzheimer's disease. People who inherit two copies of the apoE-4 gene have an eight times greater risk of developing Alzheimer's than those with the apoE-3 pair; centenarians rarely have an apoE-4 gene. The luckiest people are those who inherit one or two of the apoE-2 genes—they have the lowest risk of Alzheimer's.

While apoE genes represent one of the strongest links to an age-related disease, they remain a puzzle. Researchers don't know why the apoE-4 gene greatly increases the risk of Alzheimer's, nor why apoE-2 seems to protect against it. The protection conferred by apoE-2 and apoE-3 appears to come from their ability to bind to the amyloid beta protein and remove it from brain cells. When amyloid beta proteins are not removed from the brain in a timely manner, they can pile up and cause the destruction that leads to Alzheimer's disease. Detection of these wrecked proteins in the brains of people with Alzheimer's is so far the only way to make a definitive diagnosis—but it can only be done after death.

ApoE-4's link to Alzheimer's disease may be its inability to remove amyloid beta from the brain. The resulting buildup of amyloid sludge becomes a focal point of free radical crossfire, which damages nearby brain cells. Once further research elucidates the precise mechanism of destruction in Alzheimer's disease, new therapies can be devised to control or prevent it. Large doses of vitamin E have already been shown to slow the progression of the memory-robbing disorder and doctors are prescribing it to their at-risk patients.

Just as some genes delay aging, others hasten it. People afflicted with a relatively rare disorder known as Werner's syndrome show many signs of premature aging. They start aging in their 20s, developing white hair, wrinkles, osteoporosis, cancer and heart disease and they usually die in their 40s. The gene that causes Werner's syndrome is a mutation of a normal gene that makes an enzyme that unzips DNA during cell replication to allow for DNA repair. DNA is constantly being damaged by free radicals and, usually, the cell repairs the damage swiftly by unzipping the DNA coil, cutting out the dysfunctional DNA and replacing it with healthy DNA. In people with Werner's, this repair process is blocked, resulting in the accumulation of damaged DNA and subsequent rapid appearance of age-related disorders.

The Werner's gene is just one of many that predispose people to disease. Most susceptibility genes act in more subtle ways than the Werner's gene. For example, some people possess a gene that makes them prone to developing high blood pressure when they eat a high-salt diet; people without the gene can eat salt without worry. Similar genes might predispose some people to heart disease if they eat a high-fat diet or to lung cancer if they smoke cigarettes. Once they find these susceptibility genes, doctors will be able to tailor preventive therapies to each person. Lacking this genetic precision, public health experts are forced to issue broad warnings to the public to reduce their intake of salt and fat and quit smoking.

The study of menopause may also lead to a better understanding of the genetics of aging. Before the turn of the century, few women experienced menopause because they rarely lived long enough. As women are living longer and longer, menopause has become common. Researchers are trying to figure out why a woman's reproductive cycle stops in what is now mid-life and what clues menopause holds for extending the youthful years. The first indication that menopause may be genetically choreographed came from observations that women go through menopause at about the same age as their mothers.

In his study of 78 female centenarians, Harvard's Perls found that he could roughly predict if a woman would have a long life or a short one by her age when she last became pregnant: the older a woman is when she last gets pregnant without the aid of fertility treatments, the longer she will live. Older mothers do not experience menopausal changes until much later in life than average. Women who live to be 100 are four times more likely to have had children in their 40s and 50s than women who die in their 70s.

These female centenarians, Perls surmises, have longevity genes that postpone menopause and enable them to become pregnant at older ages. Their genes also slow aging, not as a primary goal but as a side effect. For example, women in their 50s whose ovaries are still functioning and producing estrogen are at reduced risk of developing heart disease, osteoporosis and Alzheimer's disease, three major age-related disorders. All of these diseases are also delayed or prevented in women who may not be endowed with longevity genes but are taking estrogen after menopause. They are giving themselves some of the protection against aging enjoyed by centenarians and they are healthier and they live longer than postmenopausal women who are not on estrogen replacement therapy.

"There is no evolutionary benefit of living to 100," Perls explains. "That some people do live longer is secondary. The key is that they have good longevity assurance genes that greatly extend their reproductive capacity. Those genes don't just shut off after a woman goes through menopause; they keep going and they're probably the genes that allow women to go on to be 100 years old."

The discovery of anti-aging genes is important because such knowledge may help level the playing field between the lucky few who inherit the genes and the rest of the population who don't. Scientists are using genetic-engineering techniques, called biopharming, to pluck these beneficial genes from human cells and splice them into animal and plant cells. Animals with human genes produce the human protein product of the genes in their milk; plants engineered to have human genes produce human proteins in their fruit or leaves. Unlimited amounts of human proteins made by the anti-aging genes can be filtered from milk or extracted from crops, making life-extension a possibility for all of us. Some of these new drugs are already on the way, including human proteins made from anti-aging genes that can be used as drugs to prevent heart disease, cancer, osteoporosis and other chronic disorders.

Drug makers have never before been able to tap into all of the body's store of chemicals in such a massive way. So far they have developed only about 400 chemical targets in the body that they can influence with drugs, and these they have usually discovered by chance. But potential drug targets have expanded enormously to about 75,000, one for each gene in the body.

"When you think about what a small number of drugs we had to work with before and where we're headed with thousands of new chemical targets, it's bound to spark a revolution in health care," says Dr. Francis Collins, director of the National Human Genome Research Institute. "Almost every pharmaceutical company now has a gene-discovery division. They see this as their future."

Genes that retard aging are turning out to have amazing powers to quash free radicals and repair the DNA damage caused by free radicals. California Institute of Technology researchers created one of these anti-aging genes in the laboratory by mutating a normal gene to make it work harder. The hyperactive gene seems to be heavily involved in boosting defenses against free radical damage. Flies with this gene mutation live 35 percent longer than usual. Such an increase in humans would be the equivalent of boosting average life expectancy in the U.S. from 76 years to 98.

Perhaps humans who live to be 100 without serious disease have similar genes that boost antioxidants or in other ways reduce free radical damage. As scientists get their hands on more of the longevity genes of centenarians, evolution will be taking a back seat to human ingenuity in driving life span to new records.

# *About the Author*

Ronald Kotulak, a *Chicago Tribune* science writer, won the Pulitzer Prize for Explanatory Journalism in 1994 for breakthrough reporting on early brain development. A past president of the National Association of Science Writers, Kotulak has won numerous national writing awards from groups that include the American Psychiatric Association, American Chemical Society, American Aging Association, American Medical Association, American Heart Association, and the National Mental Health Association. In 1995, Kotulak received the American Diabetes Association's C. Everett Koop Medal for Health Promotion and Awareness. The University of Michigan honored Kotulak with the 1978 Outstanding Achievement Award. He is the author of *Inside the Brain: Revolutionary Discoveries of How the Mind Works* (Andrews McMeel Publishing, 1996).

# *Index*

Printed in the United States
18467LVS00007B/128